Brain Cancer Therapy and Surgical Interventions

Horizons in Cancer Research
Volume 27

HORIZONS IN CANCER RESEARCH

Volume 1: Prostate Cancer
John N. Lucas (Editor)
ISBN 1-59454-100-0

Volume 2: Trends in Ovarian Cancer Research
A. P. Bardos (Editor)
ISBN 1-59454-023-3

Volume 3: Percutaneous Cryotherapy of Renal Cell Carcinoma under an Open MRI System
Junta Harada, Kazuo Miyasaka and Sajio Sumida (Editors)
ISBN 1-59454-169-8

Volume 4: Focus on Colorectal Cancer Research
Julia D. Martinez (Editor)
ISBN 1-59454-101-9

Volume 5: Focus on Leukemia Research
Rafael M. Romero (Editor)
ISBN 1-59454-093-4

Volume 6: Progress in Bladder Cancer Research
A. M. Mallory (Editor)
ISBN 1-59454-129-9

Volume 7: Trends in Prostate Cancer Research
John N. Lucas (Editor)
ISBN 1-59454-265-1

Volume 8: Tumor Budding in Colorectal Cancer Recent Progress in Colorectal Cancer Research
Tadahiko Masaki (Editor)
ISBN 1-59454-189-2

Volume 9: Trends in Breast Cancer Research
Andrew P. Yao (Editor)
ISBN 1-59454-134-5

Volume 10: Trends in Leukemia Research
Rafael M. Romero (Editor)
ISBN 1-59454-311-9

Volume 11: Liver Cancer: New Research
Felix Lee (Editor)
ISBN 1-59454-182-5

Volume 12: Focus on Lung Cancer
Robert L. Carafaro (Editor)
ISBN 1-59454-082-9

Volume 13: Treatment of Ovarian Cancer
A. P. Bardos (Editor)
ISBN 1-59454-022-5

Volume 14: Focus on Kidney Cancer Research
Kelvin R. Nunez (Editor)
ISBN 1-59454-110-8

Volume 15: Focus on Pacreatic Cancer Research
Maxwell A. Loft (Editor)
ISBN 1-59454-270-8

Volume 16: Peritoneal Carinomatosis from Ovarian Cancer
Kostantinos N. Chatzigeorgiou and John N. Bontis (Editors)
ISBN 1-59454-398-4

Volume 17: Trends in Pacreatic Cancer Research
Maxwell A. Loft (Editor)
ISBN 1-59454-524-3

Volume 18: Trends in Kidney Cancer Research
Kelvin R. Nunez (Editor)
ISBN 1-59454-141-8

Volume 19: Ovarian Cancer: New Research
A. P. Bardos (Editor)
ISBN 1-59454-241-4

Volume 20: Gene Therapy in Cancer
Grace W. Redberry (Editor)
ISBN 1-59454-288-0

Volume 21: Lung Cancer New Research
Robert L. Carafaro (Editor)
ISBN 1-59454-

Volume 22: New Developments in Bone Cancer Research
Catherine E. O'Neil (Editor)
ISBN 1-59454-337-2

Volume 23: New Developments in Breast Cancer Research
Andrew P. Yao (Editor)
ISBN 1-59454-809-9

Volume 24: Trends in Bone Cancer Research
E. V. Birch (Editor)
ISBN 1-59454-346-1

Volume 25: Focus on Brain Cancer Research
Andrew V. Yang (Editor)
ISBN 1-59454-973-7

Volume 26: Cancer Vaccine: New Research
(Editor)
ISBN 1-59454-968-0

Volume 27: Brain Cancer Therapy and Surgical Interventions
Andrew V. Yang (Editor)
ISBN 1-59454-974-5

Brain Cancer Therapy and Surgical Interventions

Horizons in Cancer Research
Volume 27

Andrew V. Yang
Editor

Nova Biomedical Books
New York

For permission to use material from this book please contact us:
Telephone 631-231-7269; Fax 631-231-8175
Web Site: http://www.novapublishers.com

Library of Congress Cataloging-in-Publication Data

Brain cancer therapy and surgical interventions / Andrew V. Yang, editor.
p. ; cm.
Includes bibliographical references and index.
ISBN 1-59454-974-5
1. Brain--Cancer--Chemotherapy. 2. Brain--Cancer--Surgery. I. Yang, Andrew V.
[DNLM: 1. Brain Neoplasms--drug therapy. 2. Brain Neoplasms--surgery. WL 358 B8128 2006]
RC280.B7B73 2006
616.99'48106--dc22 2006000905

Published by Nova Science Publishers, Inc. ✢New York

Contents

Preface

There are two types of brain tumors: primary brain tumors that originate in the brain and metastatic (secondary) brain tumors that originate from cancer cells that have migrated from other parts of the body. Primary brain cancer rarely spreads beyond the central nervous system, and death results from uncontrolled tumor growth within the limited space of the skull. Metastatic brain cancer indicates advanced disease and has a poor prognosis. Primary brain tumors can be cancerous or noncancerous. Both types take up space in the brain and may cause serious symptoms (e.g., vision or hearing loss) and complications (e.g., stroke). All cancerous brain tumors are life threatening (malignant) because they have an aggressive and invasive nature. A noncancerous primary brain tumor is life threatening when it compromises vital structures (e.g., an artery). In the United States, the annual incidence of brain cancer generally is 15-20 cases per 100,000 people. Brain cancer is the leading cause of cancer-related death in patients younger than 35. This new book brings together the leading research in this dynamic area of research.

Most antitumor drugs are excluded from the brain by a series of physiological barrier between the blood and the central nervous system (CNS) microenvironment. These barriers arise from unique properties of CNS blood vessel endothelial cells and specialized epithelial cells. Both of the cell types utilize tight junctions to prevent bulk flow of blood-born products into the brain. Overcoming the limitations imposed by the blood-brain barrier is critical to achieving therapeutic concentrations of drugs in the CNS, and has been the focus of intense research. Chapter 1 discusses past, present, and future approaches to manipulating the blood-brain barriers and reviews the most effective ways of delivering drugs in order to improve the outcome of patients with malignant brain tumors.

Despite recent advances in surgical technology, many brain stem tumors, mainly diffuse pediatric gliomas, have been regarded as inoperable until today. Local drug delivery approaches to this eloquent area have therefore gained increasingly research interest. First experiments have been performed on rodents. Chapter 2 describes the current experimental efforts and latest laboratory findings concerning local drug infusion systems for the brain stem. The English-language literature on brain stem tumor models and therapy approaches for local drug delivery by infusion systems was reviewed using the MEDLINE Pub Med database (1966-present). Current concepts, drug delivery methods (high-flow and low-flow), animal models (rats, mice, monkeys), pharmacokinetic, radiologic and histologic data of drug distribution as well as clinical data of side effects such as neurotoxicity are presented. Catheter implantation into the brainstem of animals for the purpose of drug delivery appears to be safely possible. On the basis of the currently available data, chronic drug delivery of certain agents seems to be tolerated in different animals in potentially effective doses. Clinico-neurological side effects are dose- and drug dependent and showed variability even in the same kind of animals. Local drug infusion systems will most likely become an important mechanism for drug delivery to the brainstem in the future. The preliminary findings have layed the groundwork for further investigations and give the hope for clinical trials in the future.

Substance P is an undecapeptide that belongs to the tachykinin family of peptides and has a widespread distribution in both the central and peripheral nervous systems. It is known that substance P, neurokinin A, neuropeptide K and neuropeptide Gamma are derived from the preprotachykinin A gene, whereas neurokinin B is derived from the preprotachykinin B gene. The biological actions of substance P, neurokinin A and neurokinin B are mediated by three receptors, designated neurokinin (NK)-1, NK-2 and NK-3, the biological action of substance P being preferentially mediated by the NK1 receptor. After binding to the NK1 receptor, substance P regulates many biological functions, and this neuropeptide has also been implicated in inflammation, pain and depression. Preclinical investigations have shown that activation of the NK1 receptor by substance P induces mitogenesis in several human tumour cell lines, and that NK1 receptor antagonists (e.g., L-733,060) display antitumoural action against human cancer cell lines (glioma, retinoblastoma, neuroblastoma…). In addition, it has been documented that astrocytomas and gliomas contain significant levels of NK1 receptors and that both express substance P. Thus, the development of antagonist molecules of the NK1 receptor represents an important opportunity for exploiting these molecules as novel therapeutic agents. The antitumoural action of one of these antagonists (L-733,060) (estimated affinity = 0.8 nM) has been tested in several cancer cell lines (glioma, neuroblastoma, retinoblastoma…), but the antitumoural action of other NK1 receptor antagonists (e.g., L-732,138) is unknown. Accordingly, the aim chapter 3, using the tetrazolium compound [3-(4,5-dimethylthiazol-2-yl)-5-(3-carboxymethoxyphenyl)2-(4-sulfophenyl)-2H-tetrazolium], inner salt, a colorimetric method to evaluate cell viability, was to demonstrate the antitumoural action of the potent and highly selective competitive NK1 receptor antagonist L-732,138 (N-acetyl-L-tryptophan 3, 5-bis(trifluoromethyl) benzyl ester) (IC_{50} = 2.3 nM) on the GAMG glioma cell line and compare its antitumoural action with those previously reported in the same tumour cell line after using the selective, potent and long-acting non-peptide tachykinin NK1 receptor antagonist L-733,060. In addition, here we review the data currently available about the action of substance P and NK1 receptor antagonists in human cancer cell lines (glioma, astrocytoma, retinoblastoma…). The following aspects are discussed: 1) Substance P and the NK1 receptor; 2) Mitogenic action of substance P; 3) NK1 receptor antagonists; 4) Antitumoural action of L-732,138 on the human GAMG glioma cell line; 5) Antitumoural action of NK1 receptor antagonists; 6) Substance P, inflammation, pain and cancer; 7) Substance P, psychiatric disorders and cancer: possible relationship between the progression of cancer and cerebral mechanisms; 8) Possible clinical implications of NK1 receptor antagonists; 9) Future research on NK1 receptor antagonists. The data suggest that NK1 receptor antagonists act as a broad-spectrum antitumoural agent and that they could be a promising therapeutic drug for the treatment of human brain tumours.

Therapeutic agents affecting specific targets in cancer cells have begun to occupy an important position in cancer treatment. These treatments, known as targeted therapies, exert their effect via two main mechanisms. One group of these therapeutic agents is monoclonal antibodies which block receptors on the cell surface, deliver anti-neoplastic agents or facilitate the immune response. A second group of agents are small molecules which enter the cell and interrupt signaling pathways necessary for cancerous growth. Several drugs which affect single targets are used successfully for malignancies outside the brain in oncological practice. Imatinib mesylate, gefitinib, erlotinib, bevacizumab, inhibitors of farnesyltransferase and multitargeted agents such as antineoplastons (ANP) are also being used in extensive clinical studies in neuro-oncology. Imatinib, gefitinib and erlotinib do not appear to have antitumor activity in high-grade gliomas as single agents, but may produce a synergistic effect with chemotherapy. ANP shows promising results in phase II studies of high and low grade gliomas, brain stem gliomas and a number of responses in preliminary reports in primitive neuroectodermal tumors, atypical teratoid/rhabdoid tumors and multicentric gliomas. The efficacy of these agents has not yet been confirmed in phase III studies. Chapter 4 reviews the most important molecular targets, mechanisms of action and results of clinical trials of new generation of antineoplastic drugs that selectively destroy neoplastic cells in brain tumors.

The development of cancer treatments with better outcomes and longer survival times continues to increase the chance of encountering metastatic brain tumors. Tumor removal by craniotomy and adjuvant whole brain radiotherapy (WBRT) are common methods of treatment, and stereotactic radiosurgery such as gamma knife radiosurgery (GKS) has recently become widely used as reported in chapter 5. The major advantages of GKS are low invasiveness, short duration of hospitalization, effect independent of tumor histology, and repeatability. Deep-seated lesions in locations such as the brain stem are also good candidates for GKS. In addition, GKS is effective against metastatic brain tumors from radioresistant cancers such as renal cell carcinoma or malignant melanoma. Although good tumor growth control rate and low incidence of local recurrence have been reported, there is no prophylactic effect against the further development of new tumors. This disadvantage is overcome by the repeatability of GKS, which can be used to treat newly developed metastases following the first GKS. The optimum treatment for multiple metastatic brain tumors remains controversial. WBRT is standard, but more than 10-20 metastases can only be treated by GKS if the tumor diameters are less than 1 cm. On the other hand, WBRT is still important in the strategy for numerous metastases or metastatic cerebrospinal dissemination. Median survival time of patients who received GKS for metastatic brain tumors is less than 1 year, and more than 70% of patients died of systemic progression of the primary malignancy, not the brain metastases. Therefore, the goal of treatment by GKS is to avoid neurogenic death and to maintain good activity in daily life, not to achieve longer survival time. Radiosurgery should be considered as the optimum treatment modality for patients with brain metastases if the primary or distant metastases are well controlled, even if the lesions are multiple or newly developed after initial GKS.

Primary central nervous system neoplasm's (CNS) are the most frequent solid tumors in childhood. Despite developments in neurosurgery, radiotherapy and chemotherapy, a significant proportion of these patients suffer progressive disease. A good treatment management strategy should consider not only survival but also the quality of life of the child. Irradiation is an essential part in the management of the majority of CNS tumors. During the last decade, there were significant advances in the technology of planning and delivery of radiation treatment. Conformal radiotherapy techniques are performed using multiple treatment fields; each shaped to conform to the beam's eye view of the target volume. It allows a high homogenous dose to the tumor region with minimizing doses to normal tissue. This is particularly important for children with localized low-grade tumors, whose prognosis of long- term survival is often excellent and should be accompanied by smallest possible risk of the treatment toxicity. Many reports stress the impact of radiotherapy technical quality on survival. In our report the protracted irradiation and correctness of whole brain fields may be a major contributing factor for the overall outcome in children with medulloblastoma. The new approach of radiotherapy such a conformal, intensity modulated photon beam and stereotactic methods have recently been developed. These new methods in therapy of pediatric brain tumors and our experience in treatment of children with medulloblastoma, low-grade astrocytoma, craniopharyngioma and brain stem tumors are presented. Chapter 6 summarizes therapeutic aspects of most childhood brain tumors.

Primary brain tumors are classified according to their predominant cell type. According to the Central Brain Tumor Registry of the United States (CBTRUS), glial neoplasms are the most common primary intracranial malignancies. Although the use of SRS for well-defined small low-grade tumors is appealing, the data regarding the use of SRS is limited and insufficient to support a standard role for SRS in the initial management of low-grade gliomas. As reported in chapter 7, the technologies of F-SRT will slowly be integrated into conventional therapy, treatment margins will be reduced and SRS will be limited to very selected recurrent tumors.

In: Brain Cancer Therapy and Surgical Interventions... ISBN 1-59454-974-5
Editor: Andrew V. Yang, pp. 1-23

Chapter I

Overcoming the Barriers of the Central Nervous System: Novel Methods of Drug Delivery to Brain Cancer

Adam M. Schmitt and Maciej S. Lesniak*

The University of Chicago Pritzker School of Medicine, Chicago, IL

Abstract

Most antitumor drugs are excluded from the brain by a series of physiological barrier between the blood and the central nervous system (CNS) microenvironment. These barriers arise from unique properties of CNS blood vessel endothelial cells and specialized epithelial cells. Both of the cell types utilize tight junctions to prevent bulk flow of blood-born products into the brain. Overcoming the limitations imposed by the blood-brain barrier is critical to achieving therapeutic concentrations of drugs in the CNS, and has been the focus of intense research. This chapter discusses past, present, and future approaches to manipulating the blood-brain barriers and reviews the most effective ways of delivering drugs in order to improve the outcome of patients with malignant brain tumors.

Introduction

The American Cancer Society estimates that approximately 18,500 new cases of brain tumors will be diagnosed in 2005, 20-25% of which are projected to be of the most aggressive type, glioblastoma multiforme. Conventional treatment of glioblastoma

* To Whom Correspondence Should Be Addressed. Section of Neurosurgery, The University of Chicago Pritzker School of Medicine, 5841 South Maryland Ave, MC 3026, Chicago, IL 60637; Tel (773) 834-4757 Fax (773) 834-2608; Email: mlesniak@surgery.bsd.uchicago.edu

multiforme includes surgical resection to relieve mass effect, and subsequent radiotherapy to prolong survival. With surgery alone median survival is six months, and subsequent radiotherapy merely extends it to nine months [1, 2]. Unfortunately, most systemically administered chemotherapeutic agents are effectively excluded from the CNS, and consequently are ineffective in the treatment of brain neoplasms. However, recent scientific and technologic advances have led to the development of new, more potent antineoplastic agents as well as drug delivery systems that can help these agents reach tumors within the brain.

CNS Barriers to Drug Treatments

In contrast to systemic tissues which are freely perfused by blood, CNS parenchyma is shielded from the chemical environment of the blood by specialized protective organs, which allow essential chemicals to pass through while excluding nearly everything else. In the normal CNS, two unique organs contribute to this barrier: the blood-brain barrier (BBB), and the blood-cerebrospinal fluid barrier (BCB). However, blood vessels in CNS tumors can develop a pathological variation of the BBB, called the blood-tumor barrier (BTB), which often differs functionally from the normal BBB. Together these three barriers regulate the entrance of materials into the CNS.

With a surface area approximately 5000 times greater than the BCB, the BBB accounts for the primary interface of molecular exchange between the blood and non-pathological CNS [3]. Central to BBB physiology, endothelial cells of normal CNS capillaries are joined together in tight junctions, preventing paracellular diffusion of blood contents. Significantly, these tight junctions remain highly amenable to modification, and are regulated directly by factors released by perivascular glial cells [4-6]. As a result of tight junctions, molecular exchange across the BBB is restricted to the transcellular route across endothelial cells. Furthermore, pinocytic activity, prevalent in systemic capillary endothelial cells, is virtually absent in endothelial cells of CNS capillaries. Consequently, penetration of hydrophilic molecules in the CNS interstitium is mediated by specific molecular transporters and channels in the endothelial cells, such as the GLUT1 glucose transporter. While these specializations of CNS vasculature restrict access of hydrophilic molecules to the CNS, lipophilic molecules are largely unregulated as they are able to diffuse through the endothelial cell membrane. One particular example of this pathway's effectiveness is illustrated by the potent action of systemically delivered heroin in the CNS. More lipophilic than other opiates, heroin easily crosses the BBB and accumulates with in the CNS, enhancing the drug's effectiveness.

A collection of proteins termed multi-drug resistant efflux pumps actively work at the endothelial cells to remove both hydrophilic and lipophilic compounds that have penetrated the BBB. This decreases the efficacy of many drugs despite their ability to penetrate the BBB [7]. One member of this class, the transmembrane ATPase transporter P-glycoprotein (PGP), is believed to be responsible for low intrathecal levels of many chemotherapeutic agents (i.e., doxorubicin, vinblastine, vincristine) despite the fact that they are lipophilic.

In addition to endothelial cells, a group of perivascular cells help to maintain the endothelium and provide a second line of defense for CNS, removing materials that successfully exited the capillary. The basal surface of the endothelial cell shares a basement membrane with perivascular astrocytes and pericytes. Perivascular astrocytes are responsible for communication between capillaries and neurons and release factors which maintain endothelial cell tight junctions, whereas pericytes and macrophages phagocytose materials which have traversed the capillary endothelium.

The BTB arises from the unique characteristics of capillaries supplying CNS tumors. Like the BBB, this organ prevents the entry of many blood-borne materials into tumor tissue. However, unlike the BBB, there exists marked heterogeneity in the cellular organization and mechanisms of barrier function within the BTB. More than thirty years ago, Long noted that the vascular endothelium of tumor cells had lost many of the specializations associated with the normal BBB. Among them, he noted wide gap junctions, abnormal perivascular glia, and an increased number of endothelial cell vesicles [8]. Presumably, these defects in the BTB are responsible for tumor enhancement seen when contrast agents are administered during MRI or CT, which are excluded by the normal BBB (Figure 1). Furthermore, tumors promote growth of new capillaries into the tumor with the release of angiogenic factors such as vascular endothelial growth factor (VEGF). Additionally, VEGF has been shown to be a potent activator of vascular permeability [9]. Tumor angiogenesis is often marked by the formation of abnormal vessel structures such as arteriovenous shunts and venous anastomoses. Irregular blood flow results from these vascular developments and, with it, increased permeability of the endothelium often leads to tumor and peritumoral edema. Consequentially, capillaries in the tumor and surrounding tissue collapse due to increased interstitial pressure, compromising blood flow and limiting the ability of drugs to reach the tumor [10].

Lastly, the BCB prevents blood products from mixing with the cerebrospinal fluid (CSF) bathing the CNS. As the specialized vascular structures of the BBB are absent at the circumventricular organs of the CNS, such as the choroid plexus and the area postrema, these organs are richly bathed in blood plasma. Surrounding these tissues, a layer of choroid epithelial cells, fused together with tight junctions, prevents passage of plasma materials from the circumventricular organs into the CNS parenchyma and the adjacent CSF. Moreover, these cells are endowed with an organic-acid transport system, providing a mechanism for active clearance of molecules out of the CSF. This organic-acid transport system is believed to be responsible for the clearance of several chemotherapies from the CSF, despite their ability to cross the BBB. Although the BCB comprises a relatively small surface area, it significantly contributes to brain homeostasis since CSF circulates throughout the CNS, exchanging molecules with the interstitial fluid of the brain parenchyma.

The considerable redundancy of barrier and clearance mechanisms across these three organs underlines both the importance of shielding normal CNS parenchyma from the insulting chemical environment of the blood and the enormous hurdle these mechanisms present in attempting to deliver effective concentrations of drugs to CNS tumors. Significantly, in attempting to disrupt the barrier to deliver drugs to the CNS, one must consider the potential side-effects of diminishing the natural ability of the brain to shield itself from chemical insults.

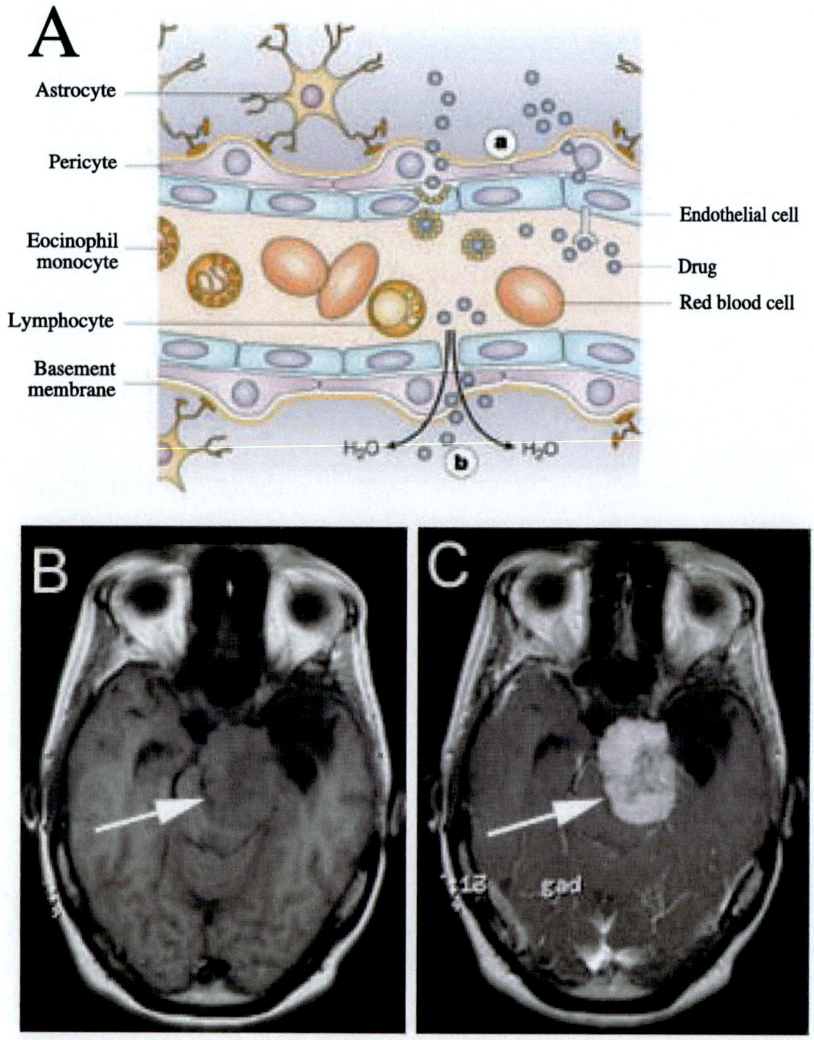

Figure 1: The blood brain barrier. A. Tight junctions between endothelial cells of CNS blood vessels prevent bulk flow of drugs into the brain from blood. Instead, endovascular drug delivery systems have focused on two mechanisms: modifying drugs to help them pass through BBB (a) and opening the BBB to allow drugs to enter the brain (b). This barrier function is often compromised in tumor vasculature. B. In this T1-weighted MRI, the tumor (arrow) is isodense to surrounding brain parenchyma. But following intravenous gadolinium infusion, the tumor tissue is perfused while the normal parenchyma surrounding the tumor has excluded the contrast agent (C). Reprinted with permission [98].

Methods of Drug Delivery to the CNS

As our understanding of the barrier mechanism in the CNS has grown, several novel approaches have been developed to overcome the limitations of drug delivery seen under intact barrier conditions. These approaches can broadly be categorized into two different classes: endovascular and surgical. Endovascular delivery systems employ cerebral blood vessels to transport drugs efficiently to many tissues throughout the brain. As the microvessels penetrate the parenchyma throughout the CNS and tumors, and at relatively short intervals, in theory drugs can be delivered throughout a tumor without concerns that the drug will have to diffuse long distances into the center of a tumor. Furthermore, as drugs are delivered throughout the CNS, there is potential to deliver drugs to wide areas of the CNS, proactively treating against tumor growth and metastases.

Endovascular approaches for drug delivery have focused on two different mechanisms of surmounting the BBB. The first of these involves mechanical or chemical disruption of the endothelium of CNS capillaries to allow drugs to enter both tumor and parenchyma. Intracarotid infusions of hyperosmolar solutions of mannitol or arabinose have been shown to disrupt the BBB and allow passage of molecules into the CNS parenchyma. Hyperosmolar solutions seem to permeabilize the capillary endothelium in two ways, first by osmotic shrinkage of endothelial cells and second by expansion of the capillary lumen as interstitial fluid accumulate in the capillary. Together, these effects result in opening of the endothelial cell tight junctions and allow for the paracellular flow of capillary materials into CNS tissues [11]. Further studies have clearly demonstrated that osmotic BBB disruption results in increased penetration of drugs in the brain parenchyma.

Unfortunately, the promising preclinical observations of osmotic BBB disruption have not translated into positive clinical outcomes. In early clinical trials, osmotic BBB disruption combined with various chemotherapies slightly increased survival of patients with primary lymphomas [12, 13]. However, these were not randomized trials. Subsequent trials have shown no increase effectiveness of chemotherapies after osmotic disruption in various grades of gliomas [14-17]. Furthermore, hyperosmolar solutions work generally throughout the CNS to disrupt the BBB and are associated with various side effects. A 1.5% increase in brain fluid is observed following osmotic disruption resulting in hemiparesis and aphasia, but usually resolves within 48 hours following treatment with dexamethasone [15]. Moreover, seizures and some chronic conditions are encountered as other blood materials including albumin enter the CNS, which may occur during transient BBB disruption [18].

A different technique to open the CNS capillary endothelium developed out of the observation that certain molecules increase permeability specifically at the site of the tumor. Certain activators of the inflammatory response such histamine and leukotrienes have been shown to increase capillary permeability for a short time [19]. Recently, a molecule, bradykinin, and its analogs, have received much attention in this area. It is believed that this molecule transiently open the BBB selectively in tumor vasculature by interacting with B2 receptors on these endothelial cells, opening tight junctions. Cereport (RMP-7), a bradykinin analog, is approximately 100 times more effective than bradykinin itself and is resistant to enzymatic degradation. Several studies have shown increased vascular permeability and enhanced drug delivery to CNS parenchyma with administration of Cereport [20-22]. While studies in rat tumor models showed significant improvement of chemotherapy efficacy when Cereport was used, a recent phase 2 clinical trial indicates that the drug did not improve carboplatin effectiveness against recurrent malignant glioma [23]. However, the authors suggest that this may be due to sub-optimal dosage of Cereport and further investigation of the drug may be warranted.

The second method currently in development to increase endovascular drug delivery to CNS tumors involves the chemical modification of drugs to promote uptake into the tumor tissue. As most chemotherapeutic drugs are large hydrophilic molecules, they are typically excluded from CNS environment by the capillary endothelium. One attempt to overcome CNS exclusion of drugs has focused on modifying known chemotherapeutic agents to make them more lipophilic. Lomustine (CCNU) and semustine (methyl-CCNU) are both examples of structurally modified carmustine (BCNU) that are more lipophilic and thus more easily traverse the BBB. Carmustine, a nitrosourea, has been shown to be moderately effective against some malignant brain tumors [24, 25]. Regrettably, clinical trials involving systemic delivery of these BCNU variants have proven to be no more effective than BCNU itself [26]. It may be the case that increased lipophilicity of nitrosoureas negatively impacts the activity of these drugs. Interestingly, some success has been observed in coupling various drugs to lipophilic carrier molecules which can traverse the BBB. Coupling to dihydropyridine has been reported to increase CNS concentrations some chemotherapeutic agents, as well as antibiotics and neurotransmitters [27].

Conjugation of drugs to BBB traversable agents has been a second area of research in developing chemically modified drugs. This involves coupling a chemotherapeutic agent to molecules that are actively transported into the CNS, such as glucose or glutamate, thereby recruiting endogenous transporters to carry drugs into the brain parenchyma. Several different ligands have been investigated as potential carrier molecules. Conjugation of model molecules to L-glutamate has been shown to increase brain to plasma drug concentration ratio significantly, indicating that conjugation of drugs to specific small molecule ligands may provide an effective means of shuttling drugs across the BBB. It is important to note, however, that the structural arrangement of these conjugations is critical, as steric hindrance of ligand-receptor binding nullifies transport into the endothelial cell [28]. Furthermore, conjugation of drugs to peptides and monoclonal antibodies has proven efficacious in aiding drug transport across the BBB, with the added potential for specifically targeting receptors in the CNS [29, 30]. One potential pitfall of this technique is that uptake of conjugate molecules into endothelial cells does not always result in transcytosis into the parenchyma, as some molecules are instead shunted to the lysosome [31].

Finally, a significant amount of research has focused on encapsulating drugs in different materials to enhance trafficking into the brain parenchyma and shield the drugs from the effects of efflux transporter drug clearance. As these materials can be quite large (up to 500 nm in diameter) a single particle can deliver many molecules of drug to the tumor or even be used to deliver genes or large proteins. One attractive method of encapsulation involves surrounding the drugs with lipids, forming a liposome. Liposomes are proposed to deliver various drugs into the CNS by passing through the lipid membrane of endothelial cell. Furthermore, additional coating of the liposome with polyethylene glycol reduces uptake of liposomes in the rough endoplasmic reticulum, thus enhancing the efficiency of drug delivery to the tumor [32]. Studies have demonstrated that these liposomes can indeed increase the concentration of intravenously administered doxorubicin and daunorubicin concentrations in CNS tumors [33, 34]. Moreover, several clinical trials of liposome encapsulated drugs have shown the efficacy of this system in a variety of CNS tumors [35-38]. While these trials utilized simple liposomes, a new generation of targeted liposomes is in development. Fusion of various proteins and antibodies, such as apolipoprotein-E (ApoE) and mAb against the transferrin receptor, to the liposome surface are providing greater penetration of liposomes into CNS capillary endothelial cells as well as means for targeting liposomes to specific tissues.

Similar to liposomes, nanoparticles are under development as another system of large particle mediated drug delivery. Most nanoparticles are formed from poly(butyl)cyano-acrylate (PBCA) and drugs are incorporated either during PBCA polymerization or are coated onto the polymerized particle. Following drug loading, these nanoparticles are coated with polysorbated-80, which confers a lipid shell. As polysorbate-80 coated nanoparticles are administered intravenously, ApoE and various other plasma proteins are absorbed onto the particle surface. It is the addition of ApoE molecules that facilitates nanoparticle uptake by endothelial cells. ApoE interaction with LDL receptors initiates LDL-like cellular uptake of the nanoparticles. One study indicated that brain concentrations of doxorubicin can be increased 60-fold with delivery in polysorbate-coated nanoparticles [39]. Recently it was shown that polysorbate-coated nanoparticles loaded with doxorubicin are effective in a rat model of glioblastoma, significantly increasing long term survival [40]. However, it is now clear that the coating formulation of these nanoparticles is critical, as a recent study showed that polyethylene glycol-coated poly(hexadecyl)cyanoacrylate nanoparticles loaded with doxorubicin accumulate large amounts of plasma proteins and were unable to reach therapeutic concentrations in the CNS. Other surfactants were unable to preferentially bind ApoE over other plasma proteins [41]. It seems that polyethylene glycol-coated nanoparticles are unable to shield the positive charge of doxorubicin and prevent interaction of these particles with excessive amounts of plasma proteins [42].

As these novel drug delivery methods have all aimed at increasing the penetration of drugs through the BBB, less attention has focused on preventing these drugs from being effluxed. Multidrug resistance proteins, such as PGP, are expressed in both tumor cells and the luminal endothelium of capillaries and actively clear many chemotherapeutic agents from the CNS environment. PGP is believed to be responsible for the decreased brain concentrations of many lipophilic molecules. In fact, the drug vinblastine accumulated up to 46-fold higher concentrations in the CNS of PGP knockout mice than wild type counterparts [43]. Given these observations, PGP inhibition seems an attractive addition to the repertoire of chemotherapies. Unfortunately, early clinical trials of the PGP inhibitors (verapamil and cyclosporine A) were disappointing. Since then, several new PGP inhibitors, with greatly decrease systemic toxicities, have been formulated. One of these, elacridar, was able to increase brain concentrations of the drug paclitaxel to 90% of the level seen in PGP knockout mice [44]. However, PGP knockout mice are highly sensitive to neurotoxins such as ivermectine, illustrating the protective function of PGP and other multidrug resistance efflux pumps in BBB function. Therefore, the positive effects of diminishing PGP mediated drug clearance must be calculated against the risks of diminishing the integrity of the brain's protective barrier.

Unfortunately, many of these endovascular drug delivery systems are plagued by the complex, heterogeneous anatomical and physiological properties of the BTB, which result in non-uniform uptake of drugs into the tumor. While preclinical studies have demonstrated that these techniques can increase penetration of drugs into the brain parenchyma, they have not translated into clinically successful treatment regimens for CNS tumors. In light of these complications, several surgical techniques have been developed to bypass the BBB and BTB and thus, aim to deliver drugs directly to the tumor. While different systems of direct drug delivery have encountered problems of drug penetration deep into the surrounding parenchyma, as they rely on simple diffusion, a new system in development, convection-enhanced drug delivery, is using pressure gradients to drive drugs deep into the CNS parenchyma.

Bypassing the Blood-Brain Barrier

While endovascular approaches have focused on manipulating the properties of the BBB to grant access of drugs to brain tissue, various other methods involve surgical placement of devices into the tumor bed, delivering drugs locally. With these methods, the BBB is bypassed and drugs are delivered from sources which are directly in contact with the tumor. The drug, released from a local source, passes into the tumor tissue by passive diffusion down a concentration gradient. Critically, properties of the drug are crucial in determining how successfully the drug will diffuse into the tissue, with small molecular weight, neutral charged, lipophilic molecules having the fastest rate of diffusion. Furthermore, these schemes offer the benefit of reduced systemic toxicity. As many antineoplastic agents reach toxic levels systemically before high enough concentration are obtained in the CNS for efficacious drug activity, systemic administration is precluded. Although carmustine has been shown to be moderately effective against brain tumors, intravenous delivery results in short drug half-life (15 min.) with severe side effects such as pulmonary fibrosis and myelosuppression. Naturally, local drug delivery is an attractive alternative, allowing for therapeutic levels of drugs without systemic toxicity.

One of the first local drug delivery system envisioned relies on placement of a catheter directly into the tumor bed to introduce drugs. The Ommaya reservoir was initially developed in 1963 for treatment of cryptococcal meningitis. Originally the device was used to provide continuing access to ventricular space for infusion of CSF with various drugs. However, current use of this device in CNS tumors involves placement of the catheter directly into the tumor, as agents delivered into the CSF are removed from the CNS rather quickly by CSF circulation. Over the years, Ommaya reservoirs have been used to infuse various chemotherapeutic and biological agents with several case reports indicating efficacious drug delivery. However, the Ommaya reservoir delivers drugs transiently in a bolus manner rather than continuously, and has not been the subject of a large clinical trial. Since the development of the Ommaya reservoir, several new technologies have been developed which improve upon the original concept. These implantable pumps include the Infusaid pump, MiniMed PIMS pump, and the Medtronic SynchroMed system and infuse drugs at a constant rate over a long period of time. A recent study utilized an osmotic minipump to deliver two peptides intratumorally, human hemopexin fragment of MMP-2 and COOH-terminal fragment of platelet factor-4 [45]. Intratumoral administration was superior to systemic delivery and significantly inhibited growth of malignant glioma graft in mice.

Drug loaded polymers emerged as an alternative to catheter placement for local drug delivery with the development of the ethylene vinyl acetate copolymer (EVAc) by Langer and Folkman in 1976 [46]. Drugs stored in the polymer are released by diffusion through a complex network of interconnecting pores, which are large enough to accommodate macromolecules such as proteins. The EVAc polymer has been approved for use in glaucoma, asthma, diabetes, and contraceptive therapies. However, utilization of this initial polymer formulation has been restricted as the polymer is non-biodegradable, and it remains in the tissue as a foreign body following drug delivery.

Second generation polymer formulations have overcome the limitations of EVAc. Various polymer formulations have been developed that are biodegradable, which release drugs both through diffusion out of the polymer and via polymer breakdown (Figure 2). One example of the second generation polymers, polyanhydride poly[bis(p-carboxyphenoxy)propane-sebacic acid] or PCPP-SA, readily reacts with water, and breaks down to dicarboxylic acids, and is neither cytotoxic, mutagenic, nor teratogenic [47, 48]. Furthermore, as the polymer is hydrophobic, water can only access the surface of the polymer, with polymer degradation occurring in a process known as surface erosion. Polymer hydrophobicity also shields the drug from interaction with the interstitial fluid, which may result in drug degradation. In addition, the specific ratio of CPP to SA in the copolymer formulation determines the rate of erosion, and can accommodate a great range of breakdown rates. For instance, 1mm thick wafer of 20% CPP/80% SA will completely erode in three weeks, whereas 100% CPP would require three years. Moreover, PCPP-SA copolymers can be produced in a variety of shapes and sizes.

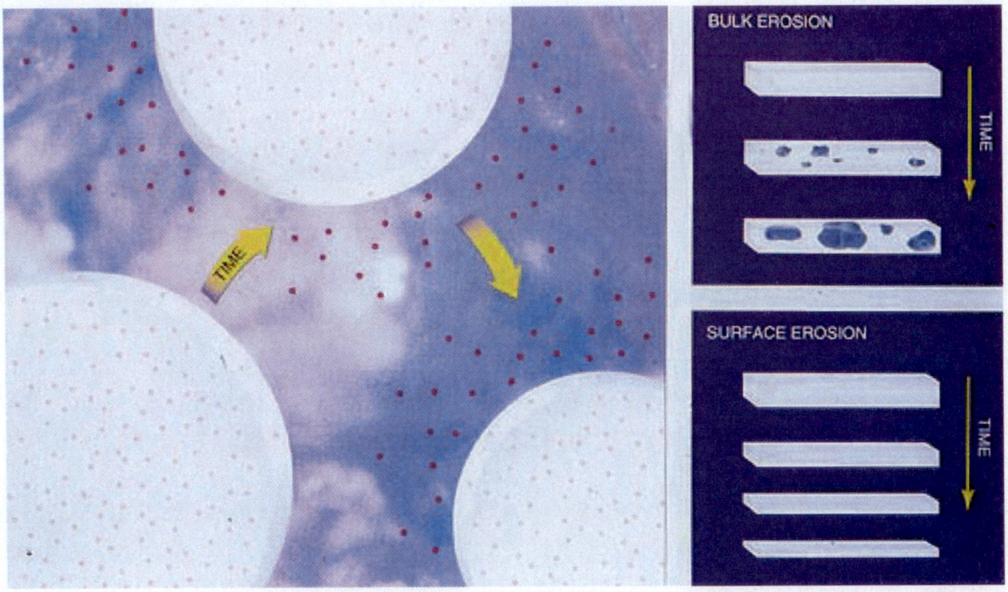

Figure 2: Biodegradable controlled release polymer implants are intended to release their drug content at a nearly constant rate as they dissolve in body water, as depicted in the large illustration. Their desirable properties therefore include surface erosion rather than bulk erosion and release of drug by degradation rather than by diffusion. These properties are shown schematically in the smaller diagrams and depend on the nature of the chemical bonds in the polymer. Reprinted with permission [99].

Despite many advantages over earlier EVAc copolymers, PCPP-SA copolymers have been limited in their ability to release, and thus efficaciously deliver some hydrophilic compounds, including hydrolytic chemotherapeutic agents such as carboplatin and methotrexate. This limitation spurred the development of new biodegradable polymers. One such system, the fatty acid dimmer-sebacic acid (FAD-SA) copolymer can be formed into different shapes and erosion rates vary with the ratio of FAD to SA, similar to PCPP-SA. However, unlike PCPP-SA copolymers, FAD-SA can reliably deliver various hydrophilic compounds, including carboplatin and proteins [49, 50]. Several other polymer formulations have been developed to deliver various drugs, including anthracyclines and cytokines, as well as the radiosensitive chemical 5-flourouracil, and in one example, polymer microspheres were applied stereotactically to the brain [51-53].

Development of Gliadel®

The development of biodegradable polymers as a method of local drug delivery opened a promising avenue of new chemotherapeutics research. As local delivery of chemotherapeutic agents avoids toxicity associated with systemic delivery of many of these agents, a broad spectrum of antineoplastic agents became candidates for delivery with this new technology. Although BCNU was known to be moderately effective against malignant brain tumors, systemic toxicity precluded intravenous delivery of the drug, making it an attractive candidate for local delivery within the brain tumor cavity. Furthermore, BCNU's characteristic small molecular weight and moderate lipid solubility made it compatible with PCPP-SA polymers, both because of its ability to be released from this polymer formulation and diffuse through tissue. For these reasons, BCNU was chosen for the initial trials of polymer mediated chemotherapy delivery in the CNS.

In preclinical studies of BCNU administration from PCPP-SA polymer in rabbits, the drug was observed to have penetrated well into surrounding parenchyma, achieving BCNU concentrations of 6mM at a distance of 10mm from the wafer within one week [54]. Furthermore, *in vitro* and *in vivo* assays of BCNU activity indicated the drug remained effective after release from the polymer. Initial studies in a rat 9L glioma model demonstrated increased efficacy of local polymer-mediated BCNU delivery over systemic BCNU [55]. In fact, the polymer method extended survival of these animals by more than two fold over systemically delivered BCNU. Moreover, BCNU polymers were well tolerated in primate studies of drug toxicity [56]. Given these promising early studies, the drug formulation entered clinical trials.

Twenty-one patients with recurrent unilateral malignant gliomas were enrolled in the initial phase I/II clinical trial of Gliadel® [57]. In this trial, up to eight drug-loaded polymers, consisting of 1.93%, 3.85%, or 6.35% BCNU by weight, were placed in the tumor cavity (Figure 3). No patients developed signs of either systemic or local toxicity. Having proven the safety of the treatment, the trial entered phase III. Two hundred twenty-two patients with recurrent malignant gliomas were enrolled in this prospective, double-blind trial comparing the effect of 3.85% BCNU loaded PCPP-SA polymers with placebo control [58]. Patients in the both groups were similar in age and tumor histology, and all had a Karnofsky performance score greater than 60, indicating independent function. While the median survival of patients who received placebo implants was 23 weeks, patients that received 3.85% BCNU loaded polymers had a median survival of 31 weeks (Figure 4) (hazard ratio = 0.69, p = 0.005). Having shown that BCNU polymers were safe and effective in the treatment of recurrent malignant gliomas, Gliadel® received FDA approval in 1996 and was the first new treatment approved for malignant brain tumors in 23 years.

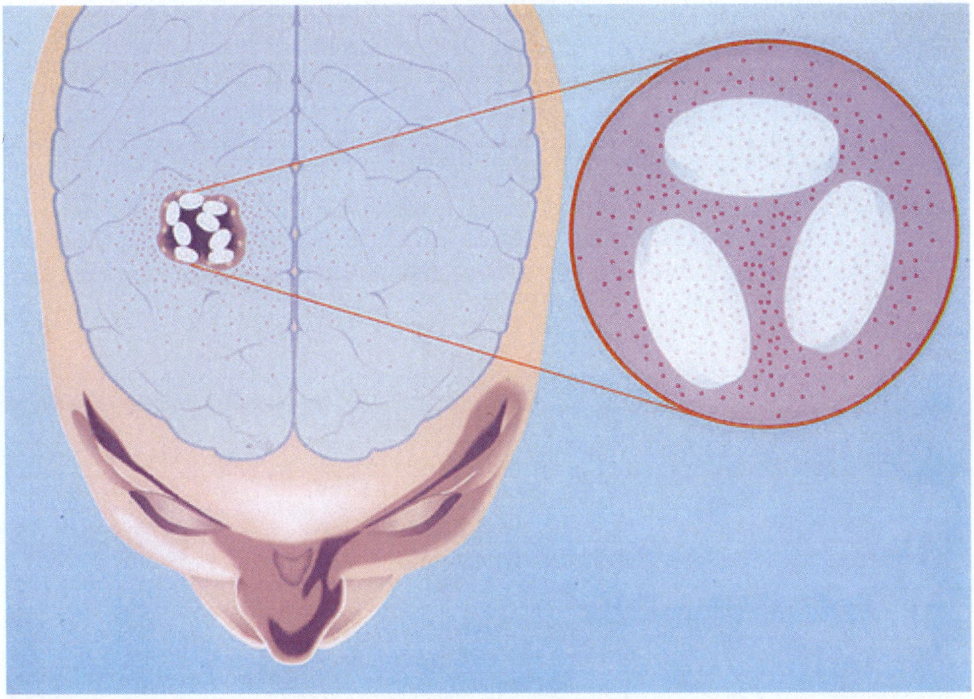

Figure 3: Up to eight polymer implants line the tumor resection cavity, where the loaded drug is gradually released as they dissolve. The inset shows conceptually how drug molecules diffuse away from these implants. Reprinted with permission [99].

With the demonstrated success of the Gliadel® system in the treatment of recurrent malignant tumors, further work naturally focused on the efficacy of Gliadel® in the initial treatment of these tumors. A prospective, double-blind phase III trial compared the effect of 3.85% BCNU polymers against placebo implanted in the tumor cavity following resection of newly diagnosed malignant glioma [59]. In this study, all patients received post-operative external beam radiation in addition to the polymer. Patients receiving 3.85% BCNU loaded polymers showed a median survival of 13.9 months whereas the median survival of placebo treated patients was 11.6 months, with a 28% (p= 0.03) reduction of risk of death. Profoundly, the Gliadel® treatment group showed 3 year survival of 9.2%, compared to just 1.7% in placebo controls. Moreover, the BCNU treatment resulted in statistically significant increase in time to decline of most measurements of the Karnofsky performance status. Based on these results, FDA approval of Gliadel® was extended to the treatment of malignant gliomas after initial resection.

Table 1. Summary of Drug/Polymer Combinations Tested in Animal Models of Malignant

Polymer/Drug Formulation	Chemotherapeutic activity of Drug	Extension of Medial Survival in F98 or 9L Glioma Model	Refs.
pCPP:SA (20:80)/3.85% BCNU	DNA Alkylation	127%	[82]
pCPP:SA (20:80)/20% BCNU	DNA Alkylation	>1,200%	[82]
pCPP:SA (20:80)/20% Taxol	Inhibitor of Microtubule Depolymerization	215%	[83]
pCPP:SA (20:80)/50% Campothecin	Inhibitor of DNA Topoisomerase 1	306%	[84]
pCPP:SA (20:80)/5% Adriamycin	Intercalation into DNA Resulting in Strand Breakage	137%	[85]
pCPP:SA (20:80)/5% Carboplatin	Interstrand Cross-linking DNA		[86]
pCPP:SA (20:80)/1,25 D3 analogs	Angiogenesis Inhibitor, Upregulation of Cell Cycle Control Proteins		
pCPP:SA (20:80)/IUdr	Radiosensitization Following Incorporation into DNA		[87]
pCPP:SA (20:80)/50% Minocycline	Angiogenesis Inhibitor	200% with IP BCNU	[88]
EVAc/50% Minocycline	Angiogenesis Inhibitor	331% with IP BCNU	[84]
pCPP:SA (20:80)/5% Mitoxantrone	Inhibitor of Tumor Angiogenesis	79%	[89]
pCPP:SA (20:80)/10% Mitoxantrone	Inhibitor of Tumor Angiogenesis	163%	[89]
EVAc/33% Mitoxantrone	Inhibitor of DNA/RNA Synthesis	141%	[90]
FAD:SA (50:50)/5-FU	Interferes with DNA Synthesis		[91]
FAD:SA (50:50)/5% Carboplatin	Interstrand Cross-linkage of DNA	150%	[49]
FAD:SA (50:50)/1% Methotrexate	Antimetabolite	140%	[92]
FAD:SA (50:50)/20% 4-HC	DNA Alkylation	121%	
FAD:SA (50:50)/20% 4-HC and BSO	DNA Alkylation and Inhibitor of Glutathione Synthesis	200%	[93]
Polymer Microspheres/IL-2	Promotes Antitumor Immune Response	100%	[94]
Microsphere Polymer/IL-2 and	Antitumor Immune Response and	152%	[95]
pCPP:SA (20:80)/10% BCNU	DNA Alkylation		

Updated with permission from [96]

Recent work has also focused on optimizing BCNU local therapy in two ways. While the Gliadel® treatments obtained FDA approval for 3.85% BCNU by weight, it remained to be seen whether higher BCNU concentrations would improve the treatment efficacy. A dose titration study of local polymer delivered BCNU related toxicity have shown 20% BCNU by weight to be the maximum-tolerated dose, with significant side effects such as seizure and brain edema resulting from higher doses [60]. With a five fold increase in the concentration of this chemotherapeutic agent, a new phase III clinical trial is underway to evaluate the efficacy of higher dose BCNU loaded polymer system. A second area of active investigation is focusing on combination therapy of BCNU with O6-benzylguanine (O6-BG), a substrate inhibitor of alkylguanine-DNA alkyltransferase (AGT). AGT activity is present in most brain tumors and works to repair DNA damaged by BCNU, thus combining BCNU and O6- BG into a single treatment seems an attractive possibility. In a rat model of malignant glioma with AGT activity, co-administration of O6-BG with local polymer-mediated BCNU treatment enhanced BCNU effectiveness and extended survival [61].

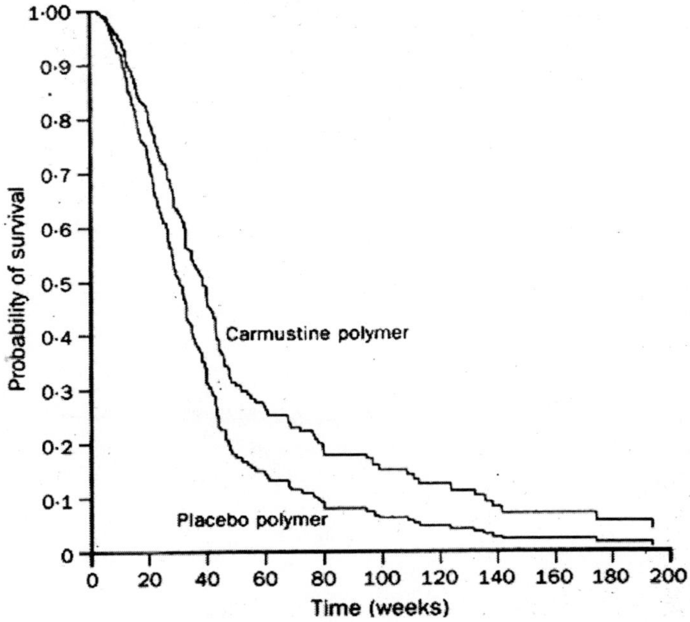

Figure 4: Overall survival for patients receiving implantation of carmustine (BCNU)-loaded polymers or placebo controls at the time of operation for a recurrent brain tumor after adjustment for prognostic factors. Reprinted with permission [58].

With the successful development of Gliadel®, polymer-mediated local drug delivery was proven as an efficacious mechanism for delivery to CNS tumors. Since then, multiple polymer formulations have been utilized to deliver different antineoplastic agents to CNS tumors (Table 1). Most of these chemotherapeutics have had limited effectiveness in the past due to systemic toxicity or inability to traverse the BBB, despite their efficacy against tumor cells *in vitro*. The polymer system has brought renewed interest into several of these chemotherapies, as well as opening the door to application of macromolecules such as IL-2 in the treatment of CNS tumors.

Microchip Delivery Systems

A significant advance in the field of local drug delivery emerged with the development in microchip drug delivery systems. These microchips consist of multiple small reservoirs etched into a silicon frame and are filled with liquid, gel, or solid and covered in a thin anode membrane (Figure 5) [62]. Electrochemical dissolution of this thin membrane releases the stored materials, and the release parameters can be modulated to allow for varied drug release profiles over extended periods of time. With up to 1000 microreservoirs in an individual chip, this technology opens the possibility for dynamic, on-demand release of various drugs locally. Furthermore, these chips can incorporate microbatteries, memory, and multiplexing circuitry, allowing for the chips to be implanted or swallowed.

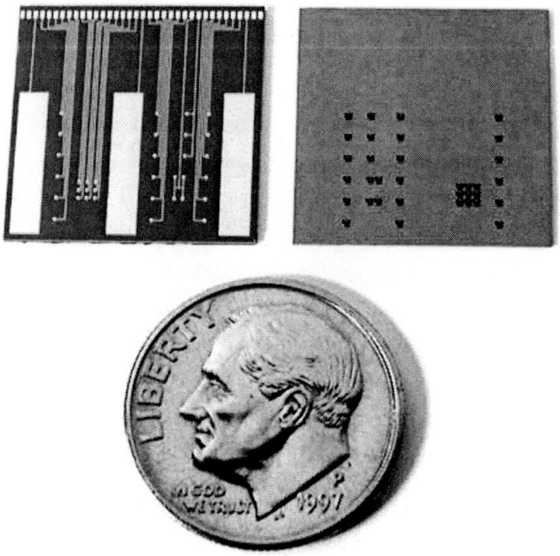

Figure 5: Microchip with dime caption. Front (left) and back views of a new microchip for the controlled release of chemicals. The dots between the three large bars (cathodes) on the front are the caps (anodes) covering the reservoirs that hold chemicals. An electrical voltage applied between a reservoir cap and a cathode causes a reaction that dissolves the cap, releasing the chemical. The back view shows the larger openings for each reservoir through which chemicals are deposited (these openings are sealed by a waterproof material after the reservoirs are filled. Photo by Paul Horwitz, Atlantic Photo Service, Inc

Beyond the original microchip design, a new generation of biodegradable microchips has been developed [63]. Rather than using electrochemical dissolution of the anode membrane to release the drugs, these chips use a biodegradable membrane to seal the reservoir. As the membrane erodes, the microreservoirs are exposed and drugs released. Moreover, the properties of the poly(D,L-lactic-co-glycolic acid) membrane can be modified to control the release parameters. Biodegradable microchips represent a promising new technology in the local delivery of drugs to CNS tumors.

Convection-Enhanced Drug Delivery

The local delivery systems outlined above all rely on drug diffusion from the source into the tumor and parenchyma, and the rate of diffusion is governed molecular weight, hydrophilicity and charge. Under these conditions, small, electrically neutral, lipophilic molecules offer the best opportunity for penetrating deep into the tissue. Unfortunately, many chemotherapeutic agents do not meet these criteria and thus their diffusion is restricted. Furthermore, large molecular weight molecules move very slowly under passive diffusion. For instance, immunoglobulin G proteins were shown to take up to three days to diffuse one millimeter into a tumor bed and normal parenchyma [64].

An alternative delivery mechanism for distributing such chemicals, convection-enhanced delivery (CED) systems utilize pressure gradients in addition to simple diffusion to drive chemicals deep into tumor and brain tissue, and have been shown to be biologically active at distant sites. Studies have demonstrated that small volumes of fluid injected into cerebral white matter create a pressure gradient which propagates the fluid across broad areas of white matter along a convection wave, without producing structural or functional damage in the surrounding tissue [65-67]. Drugs contained within the fluid are spread evenly throughout the convection area, and only after the pressure gradient is dispersed does the kinetics of drug diffusion determine the distribution. However, the volume used for white matter infusions must be restricted to a small range, if the volume is too small, the brain will clear the solution as if it were edematous fluid. But if the volume of infusion is too great, or if the rate of a continuous infusion is greater than a few microliters per minute, solution will leak out along the injection tract and the pressure gradient will be lost [65].

CED technology can also be used to specifically target drugs to discrete regions of the brain. Targeted convection-mediated delivery of an excitotoxin to the globus pallidus internus selectively ablated these neurons in a macaque monkey model of Parkinson's diseases, indicating the potential use of this technology for specifically localized delivery of cytotoxic chemical to a tumor while preserving surrounding tissue [68]. Further enhancing the ability to target specific brain regions, infusion parameters of specific tissues can be monitored non-invasively using real time, in-vivo diffusion weighted MRI imaging or CT using an iodinated tracer [69, 70]. Furthermore, DWMRI can detect different diffusion properties of tumors and potentially predict the efficacy of CED [70]. A promising recent phase I/II clinical trial of CED administered paclitaxel observed 73% of patients responding to the treatment [71]. However, the treatment was also associated with high incidence of complications, including transient neurological changes, chemical meningitis, and infection.

Beyond using CED for distributing traditional chemotherapies, an exciting application of this technology lies in the delivery of novel protein-derived therapies, such as conjugated antibodies or cytokines. The observation that glioblastoma multiforme tumor cells over-express interleukin-4 (IL-4) and interleukin-13 (IL-13) receptors opened the possibility of targeting potent therapies specifically to tumor cells by conjugating the drug to cytokines. Early studies demonstrated that both IL-4 and IL-13 conjugated Pseudomonas exotoxin (PE) specifically targeted and had potent cytotoxic activity against several glioma cell lines [72-75]. Upon binding to the IL receptor, the conjugated molecule is internalized and the ADP ribosylation activity of PE inactivates elongation factor 2, inhibiting protein synthesis and leading to cell death [76]. Both IL-4 and IL-13 conjugated PE were shown to reduce tumor size in glioma xenograft animal models, and IL13-PE showed no signs of systemic toxicity when delivered intrathecally [74, 77, 78]. Furthermore, studies of the distribution kinetics of IL13-PE have demonstrated improved penetration of the CED administered drug in tumor tissue over bolus injected drug, and prolonged presence of the drug in the tumor interstitium [79].

Based on these promising pre-clinical studies, clinical trials are underway to determine the efficacy of CED administered IL-4 and IL-13 conjugated PE. A phase I, dose-escalation clinical study has evaluated the effectiveness of IL4-PE (NBI-3001) administered by CED in patients with recurrent malignant glioma [80]. In this trial, patients received an infusion of IL4-PE from one, two, or three catheters placed intratumorally or peritumorally. The maximum tolerated dose consisted of a total infusion of 40ml of drug at concentration of 6μg/ml. Subsequent surgical resection of the tumor was performed when medically indicated. While systemic toxicity was not noted, 39% of patients experienced signs of Grade 3-4 CNS drug related toxicity, but symptoms generally were reversible. Median survival for all patients was 8.2 months, while median survival for patients with GBM was 5.8 months. Based on this work, phase II clinical trials of IL4-PE are currently underway.

In a separate phase I/II clinical trial, CED administered IL13-PE was shown to be moderately beneficial in the treatment of recurrent malignant glioma [81]. This trial established that placement of two or more catheters in the peritumor (PT) tissue improved drug dispersal to peritumor area and prolonged survival compared to intratumor (IT) catheter placement (median survivals: IT=37.1 wk, PT=44wk, ≥2 PT catheters=51.7wk). It seems that tissue heterogeneity in solid tumors decreases successful infiltration of the drug into the peritumor space when the catheter is positioned intratumorally. Furthermore, use of stereotactic catheter placement 2-4 days post-resection improved accuracy of catheter placement in the peritumor space over catheter placement immediately following resection. Following the initial success of the phase I/II trial, the PRECISE phase III clinical trial is evaluating the efficacy CED administered IL13-PE in patients with recurrent glioblastoma multiforme in comparison to local treatment with Gliadel® wafers.

Future Directions

As our understanding of the barrier function of the CNS has expanded, so to have the number of drug delivery systems which aim to overcome this barrier. While endovascular treatments offer the benefit of broad access to tissues of CNS and can be used to deliver drugs to deep tissues of the brain, many treatment paradigms have still failed to consistently deliver therapeutic doses to CNS tumors because of the mechanisms of drug exclusion and the heterogeneity of the BTB. On the other hand, surgically place local delivery devices have been successful in applying drugs directly to tumor cells, avoiding the BBB, but have been limited in their ability to access large areas of the CNS because they rely on simple diffusion into the parenchyma. Advances in drug delivery to the CNS will need to focus on optimizing and integrating the strengths of these two approaches. First, drugs must be able to overcome or bypass the BBB in order to reach tumor tissue and parenchyma. Secondly, broad distribution of the drug throughout large areas of the brain will help to proactively treat tumor expansion and metastases.

Beyond the development of new delivery mechanisms, new agents are needed that have greater activity against tumor cells. Currently, gene therapy and immunotherapy are attracting much attention as novel treatments for specifically and potently targeting CNS tumors. A promising new field of research aims to formulate viruses that specifically infect tumor cells while sparing surrounding normal cells. Moreover, the promotion of local inflammatory responses within CNS tumors using cytokines will aid the body's immune system to attack the tumor itself. Further development of these novel treatments will provide new, powerful tools against this terrible disease.

References

[1] Mohan, D.S., et al., Outcome in elderly patients undergoing definitive surgery and radiation therapy for supratentorial glioblastoma multiforme at a tertiary care institution. *Int J Radiat Oncol Biol Phys*, 1998. *42*(5): p. 981-7.

[2] Barker, F.G., et al., Survival and functional status after resection of recurrent glioblastoma multiforme. *Neurosurgery*, 1998. *42*(4): p. 709-20.

[3] Pardridge, W.M., *Blood-brain barrier transport of nutrients Fed Proc.*, 1986. *45*(7): p. 2047-9.

[4] Risau, W. and H. Wolburg, Development of the blood-brain barrier. *Trends Neurosci,* 1990. *13*(5): p. 174-8.

[5] Stannes, K.A., E. Guatteo, and D. Janigro, A dynamic model of the blood-brain barrier "in vitro". *Neurotoxicology*, 1996. *17*(2): p. 481-496.

[6] Stannes, K.A., et al., Morphological and functional characterization of an in vitro blood-brain barrier model. *Brain Res*, 1997. *771*(2): p. 329-342.

[7] Demeule, M., et al., Drug transport to the brain: key roles for the efflux pump P-glycoprotein in the blood-brain barrier. *Vascul Pharmacol*, 2002. *38*(6): p. 339-348.

[8] Long, D.M., Capillary ultrastructure and the blood-brain barrier in human malignant brain tumors. *J Neurosurg*, 1970. *32*(2): p. 127-44.

[9] Stewart, P.A., et al., Quantitative study of microvessel ultrastructure in human peritumoral brain tissue. Evidence for a blood-brain barrier defect. *J Neurosurg*, 1987. *67*(5): p. 697-705.

[10] Roose, T., et al., Solid stress generated by spheroid growth estimated using a linear poroelasticity model small star, filled. *Microvasc Res*, 2003. *66*(3): p. 204-12.

[11] Kroll, R.A. and E.A. Neuwelt, Outwitting the blood-brain barrier for therapeutic purposes: osmotic opening and other means. *Neurosurgery*, 1998. *42*(5): p. 1099-100.

[12] Doolittle, N.D., et al., Safety and efficacy of a multicenter study using intraarterial chemotherapy in conjunction with osmotic opening of the blood-brain barrier for the treatment of patients with malignant brain tumors. *Cancer*, 2000. *88*(3): p. 637-47.

[13] McAllister, L.D., et al., Cognitive outcomes and long-term follow-up results after enhanced chemotherapy delivery for primary central nervous system lymphoma. *Neurosurgery*, 2000. *46*(1): p. 51-60.

[14] Gumerlock, M.K., et al., Osmotic blood-brain barrier disruption and chemotherapy in the treatment of high grade malignant glioma: patient series and literature review. *J Neurooncol*, 1992. *12*(1): p. 33-46.

[15] Siegal, T., et al., In vivo assessment of the window of barrier opening after osmotic blood-brain barrier disruption in humans. *J Neurosurg*, 2000. *92*(4): p. 599-605.

[16] Neuwelt, E.A., et al., Therapeutic efficacy of multiagent chemotherapy with drug delivery enhancement by blood-brain barrier modification in glioblastoma. *Neurosurgery*, 1986. *19*(4): p. 573-82.

[17] Kobrinsky, N.L., et al., Etoposide with or without mannitol for the treatment of recurrent or primarily unresponsive brain tumors: a Children's Cancer Group Study, CCG-9881. *J Neurooncol*, 1999. *45*(1): p. 47-54.

[18] Nadal, A., et al., Plasma albumin is a potent trigger of calcium signals and DNA synthesis in astrocytes. *Proc Natl Acad Sci USA*, 1995. *92*(5): p. 1426-30.

[19] Connolly, D.T., Vascular permeability factor: a unique regulator of blood vessel function. *J Cell Biochem*, 1991. *47*(3): p. 219-23.

[20] Mackic, J.B., et al., Cereport (RMP-7) increases the permeability of human brain microvascular endothelial cell monolayers. *Pharm Res*, 1999. *16*(9): p. 1360-5.

[21] Emerich, D.F., et al., Enhanced delivery of carboplatin into brain tumours with intravenous Cereport (RMP-7): dramatic differences and insight gained from dosing parameters. *Br J Cancer*, 1999. *80*(7): p. 964-70.

[22] Barnett, F.H., et al., Selective delivery of herpes virus vectors to experimental brain tumors using RMP-7. *Cancer Gene Ther*, 1999. *6*(1): p. 14-20.

[23] Prados, M.D., et al., A randomized, double-blind, placebo-controlled, phase 2 study of RMP-7 in combination with carboplatin administered intravenously for the treatment of recurrent malignant glioma. *Neuro-oncol*, 2003. *5*(2): p. 96-103.

[24] Green, S.B., et al., Comparisons of carmustine, procarbazine, and high-dose methylprednisolone as additions to surgery and radiotherapy for the treatment of malignant glioma. *Cancer Treat Rep*, 1983. *67*(2): p. 121-32.

[25] Walker, M.D., et al., Randomized comparisons of radiotherapy and nitrosoureas for the treatment of malignant glioma after surgery. *N Engl J Med*, 1980. *303*(23): p. 1323-9.

[26] Kornblith, P.L. and M. Walker, Chemotherapy for malignant gliomas. *J Neurosurg*, 1988. *68*(1): p. 1-17.

[27] Prokai, L., K. Prokai-Tatrai, and N. Bodor, Targeting drugs to the brain by redox chemical delivery systems. *Med Res Rev*, 2000. *20*(5): p. 367-416.

[28] Sakaeda, T., et al., Conjugation with L-Glutamate for in vivo brain drug delivery. *J Drug Target*. 2001;9(1):23-37, 2001. *9*(1): p. 23-37.

[29] Pardridge, W., Non-invasive drug delivery to the human brain using endogenous blood-brain barrier transport systems. *Pharm. Sci. Technol*, 1999. *2*(2): p. 49-59.

[30] Zhang, Y. and W.M. Pardridge, Conjugation of brain-derived neurotrophic factor to a blood-brain barrier drug targeting system enables neuroprotection in regional brain ischemia following intravenous injection of the neurotrophin. *Brain Res*, 2001. *889*(1-2): p. 49-56.

[31] Broadwell, R.D., B.J. Balin, and M. Salcman, Transcytotic pathway for blood-borne protein through the blood-brain barrier. *Proc Natl Acad Sci USA*, 1988. *85*(2): p. 632-6.

[32] Begley, D.J., Delivery of therapeutic agents to the central nervous system: the problems and the possibilities. *Pharmacol Ther*, 2004. *104*(1): p. 29-45.

[33] Albrecht, K.W., et al., High concentration of Daunorubicin and Daunorubicinol in human malignant astrocytomas after systemic administration of liposomal Daunorubicin. *J Neurooncol*, 2001. *53*(3): p. 267-71.

[34] Koukourakis, M.I., et al., High intratumoural accumulation of stealth liposomal doxorubicin (Caelyx) in glioblastomas and in metastatic brain tumours. *Br J Cancer*, 2000. *83*(10): p. 1281-6.

[35] Lippens, R.J., Liposomal daunorubicin (DaunoXome) in children with recurrent or progressive brain tumors. *Pediatr Hematol Oncol*, 1999. *16*(2): p. 131-9.

[36] Fabel, K., et al., Long-term stabilization in patients with malignant glioma after treatment with liposomal doxorubicin. *Cancer*, 2001. *92*(7): p. 1936-42.

[37] Fiorillo, A., et al., Second-line chemotherapy with the association of liposomal daunorubicin, carboplatin and etoposide in children with recurrent malignant brain tumors. *J Neurooncol*, 2004. *66*(1-2): p. 179-85.

[38] Hau, P., et al., Pegylated liposomal doxorubicin-efficacy in patients with recurrent high-grade glioma. *Cancer*, 2004. *100*(6): p. 1199-207.

[39] Gulyaev, A.E., et al., Significant transport of doxorubicin into the brain with polysorbate 80-coated nanoparticles. *Pharm Res*, 1999. *16*(10): p. 1564-9.

[40] Steiniger, S.C., et al., Chemotherapy of glioblastoma in rats using doxorubicin-loaded nanoparticles. *Int J Cancer*, 2004. *109*(5): p. 759-67.

[41] Kreuter, J., Nanoparticulate systems for brain delivery of drugs. *Adv Drug Deliv Rev*, 2001. *47*(1): p. 65-81.

[42] Brigger, I., et al., Negative preclinical results with stealth nanospheres-encapsulated Doxorubicin in an orthotopic murine brain tumor model. *J Control Release*, 2004. *100*(1): p. 29-40.

[43] van Asperen, J., et al., Altered pharmacokinetics of vinblastine in Mdr1a P-glycoprotein-deficient Mice. *J Natl Cancer Inst*, 1996. *88*(14): p. 994-9.

[44] Kemper, E.M., et al., Modulation of the blood-brain barrier in oncology: therapeutic opportunities for the treatment of brain tumours? *Cancer Treat Rev*, 2004. *30*(5): p. 415-23.

[45] Giussani, C., et al., Local intracerebral delivery of endogenous inhibitors by osmotic minipumps effectively suppresses glioma growth in vivo. *Cancer Res*, 2003. *63*(10): p. 2499-505.

[46] Langer, R. and J. Folkman, Polymers for the sustained release of proteins and other macromolecules. *Nature*, 1976. *263*(5580): p. 797-800.

[47] Leong, K.W., B.C. Brott, and R. Langer, Bioerodible polyanhydrides as drug-carrier matrices. I: Characterization, degradation, and release characteristics. *J Biomed Mater Res*, 1985. *19*(8): p. 941-55.

[48] Leong, K.W., et al., Bioerodible polyanhydrides as drug-carrier matrices. II. Biocompatibility and chemical reactivity. *J Biomed Mater Res.* 1986 Jan;20(1):51-64, 1986. *20*(1): p. 51-64.

[49] Olivi, A., et al., Interstitial delivery of carboplatin via biodegradable polymers is effective against experimental glioma in the rat. *Cancer Chemother Pharmacol*, 1996. *39*(1-2): p. 90-6.

[50] Tabata, Y., S. Gutta, and R. Langer, Controlled delivery systems for proteins using polyanhydride microspheres. *Pharm Res*, 1993. *10*(4): p. 487-96.

[51] Menei, P., et al., Drug targeting into the central nervous system by stereotactic implantation of biodegradable microspheres. *Neurosurgery*, 1994. *34*(6): p. 1058-64.

[52] Menei, P., et al., Stereotaxic implantation of 5-fluorouracil-releasing microspheres in malignant glioma. *Cancer*, 2004. *100*(2): p. 405-10.
[53] Golumbek, P.T., et al., Controlled release, biodegradable cytokine depots: a new approach in cancer vaccine design. *Cancer Res*, 1993. *53*(24): p. 5841-4.
[54] Grossman, S.A., et al., The intracerebral distribution of BCNU delivered by surgically implanted biodegradable polymers. *J Neurosurg*, 1992. *76*(4): p. 640-7.
[55] Tamargo, R.J., et al., Interstitial chemotherapy of the 9L gliosarcoma: controlled release polymers for drug delivery in the brain. *Cancer Res*, 1993. *53*(2): p. 329-33.
[56] Brem, H., et al., Biodegradable polymers for controlled delivery of chemotherapy with and without radiation therapy in the monkey brain. *J Neurosurg*, 1994. *80*(2): p. 283-90.
[57] Brem, H., et al., Interstitial chemotherapy with drug polymer implants for the treatment of recurrent gliomas. *J Neurosurg*, 1991. *74*(3): p. 441-6.
[58] Brem, H., et al., Placebo-controlled trial of safety and efficacy of intraoperative controlled delivery by biodegradable polymers of chemotherapy for recurrent gliomas. The Polymer-brain Tumor Treatment Group. *Lancet*, 1995. *345*(8956): p. 1008-12.
[59] Westphal, M., et al., A phase 3 trial of local chemotherapy with biodegradable carmustine (BCNU) wafers (Gliadel wafers) in patients with primary malignant glioma. *Neuro-oncol*, 2003. *5*(2): p. 79-88.
[60] Olivi, A., et al., Dose escalation of carmustine in surgically implanted polymers in patients with recurrent malignant glioma: a New Approaches to Brain Tumor Therapy CNS Consortium trial. *J Clin Oncol*, 2003. *21*(9): p. 1845-9.
[61] Rhines, L.D., et al., O6-benzylguanine potentiates the antitumor effect of locally delivered carmustine against an intracranial rat glioma. *Cancer Res*, 2000. *60*(22): p. 6307-10.
[62] Santini, J.T., Jr., M.J. Cima, and R. Langer, A controlled-release microchip. *Nature*, 1999. *397*(6717): p. 335-8.
[63] Richards Grayson, A.C., et al., Multi-pulse drug delivery from a resorbable polymeric microchip device. *Nat Mater*, 2003. *2*(11): p. 767-72.
[64] Jain, R.K., Delivery of novel therapeutic agents in tumors: physiological barriers and strategies. *J Natl Cancer Inst*, 1989. *81*(8): p. 570-6.
[65] Bobo, R.H., et al., Convection-enhanced delivery of macromolecules in the brain. *Proc Natl Acad Sci USA*, 1994. *91*(6): p. 2076-80.
[66] Laske, D.W., et al., Chronic interstitial infusion of protein to primate brain: determination of drug distribution and clearance with single-photon emission computerized tomography imaging. *J Neurosurg*, 1997. *87*(4): p. 586-94.
[67] Lieberman, D.M., et al., Convection-enhanced distribution of large molecules in gray matter during interstitial drug infusion. *J Neurosurg*, 1995. *82*(6): p. 1021-9.
[68] Lonser, R.R., et al., Convection-enhanced selective excitotoxic ablation of the neurons of the globus pallidus internus for treatment of parkinsonism in nonhuman primates. *J Neurosurg*, 1999. *91*(2): p. 294-302.
[69] Croteau, D., et al., Real-time in vivo imaging of the convective distribution of a low-molecular-weight tracer. *J Neurosurg*, 2005. *102*(1): p. 90-7.

[70] Mardor, Y., et al., Monitoring response to convection-enhanced taxol delivery in brain tumor patients using diffusion-weighted magnetic resonance imaging. *Cancer Res*, 2001. *61*(13): p. 4971-3.

[71] Lidar, Z., et al., Convection-enhanced delivery of paclitaxel for the treatment of recurrent malignant glioma: a phase I/II clinical study. *J Neurosurg*, 2004. *100*(3): p. 472-9.

[72] Puri, R.K., et al., Human neurological cancer cells express interleukin-4 (IL-4) receptors which are targets for the toxic effects of IL4-Pseudomonas exotoxin chimeric protein. *Int J Cancer*, 1994. *58*(4): p. 574-81.

[73] Debinski, W., et al., Human glioma cells overexpress receptors for interleukin 13 and are extremely sensitive to a novel chimeric protein composed of interleukin 13 and pseudomonas exotoxin. *Clin Cancer Res*, 1995. *1*(11): p. 1253-8.

[74] Husain, S.R., B.H. Joshi, and R.K. Puri, Interleukin-13 receptor as a unique target for anti-glioblastoma therapy. *Int J Cancer*, 2001. *92*(2): p. 168-75.

[75] Joshi, B.H., et al., In situ expression of interleukin-4 (IL-4) receptors in human brain tumors and cytotoxicity of a recombinant IL-4 cytotoxin in primary glioblastoma cell cultures. *Cancer Res*, 2001. *61*(22): p. 8058-61.

[76] Husain, S.R. and R.K. Puri, Interleukin-13 receptor-directed cytotoxin for malignant glioma therapy: from bench to bedside. *J Neurooncol*, 2003. *65*(1): p. 37-48.

[77] Puri, R.K., et al., Preclinical development of a recombinant toxin containing circularly permuted interleukin 4 and truncated Pseudomonas exotoxin for therapy of malignant astrocytoma. *Cancer Res*, 1996. *56*(24): p. 5631-7.

[78] Husain, S.R., et al., Complete regression of established human glioblastoma tumor xenograft by interleukin-4 toxin therapy. *Cancer Res*, 1998. *58*(16): p. 3649-53.

[79] Kawakami, K., et al., Distribution kinetics of targeted cytotoxin in glioma by bolus or convection-enhanced delivery in a murine model. *J Neurosurg*, 2004. *101*(6): p. 1004-11.

[80] Weber, F., et al., Safety, tolerability, and tumor response of IL4-Pseudomonas exotoxin (NBI-3001) in patients with recurrent malignant glioma. *J Neurooncol*, 2003. *64*(1-2): p. 125-37.

[81] Prados, M., et al., Final Results of Phase I/II Studies of IL13-PE38QQR Administered Intratumorally and/or Peritumorally via Convection-Enhanced Delivery in Patients Undergoing Tumor Resection for Recurrent Malignant Glioma. Presensted at American Society of Clinical Oncology Annual Meeting, Orlando, Florida, May 2005.

[82] Sipos, E.P., et al., Optimizing interstitial delivery of BCNU from controlled release polymers for the treatment of brain tumors. *Cancer Chemother Pharmacol*, 1997. *39*(5): p. 383-9.

[83] Walter, K.A., et al., Interstitial taxol delivered from a biodegradable polymer implant against experimental malignant glioma. *Cancer Res*, 1994. *54*(8): p. 2207-12.

[84] Weingart, J.D., et al., Local delivery of the topoisomerase I inhibitor camptothecin sodium prolongs survival in the rat intracranial 9L gliosarcoma model. *Int J Cancer*, 1995. *62*(5): p. 605-9.

[85] Watts, M.C., et al., Controlled release of adriamycin in the treatment of malignant glioma. Presented at the American Association of Neurological Surgeons Annual Meeting, Dever, Colorado, April 1997.

[86] Olivi, A., et al., Direct delivery of platinum-based antineoplastics to the central nervous system: a toxicity and ultrastructural study. *Cancer Chemother Pharmacol*, 1993. *31*(6): p. 449-54.

[87] Williams, J.A., et al., Implantable biodegradable polymers for IUdR radiosensitization of experimental human malignant glioma. *J Neurooncol*, 1997. *32*(3): p. 181-92.

[88] Frazier, J.L., et al., Local delivery of minocycline and systemic BCNU have synergistic activity in the treatment of intracranial glioma. *J Neurooncol*, 2003. *64*(3): p. 203-9.

[89] DiMeco, F., et al., Local delivery of mitoxantrone for the treatment of malignant brain tumors in rats. *J Neurosurg*, 2002. *97*(5): p. 1173-8.

[90] Saini, M., et al., Intralesional mitoxantrone biopolymer-mediated chemotherapy prolongs survival in rats with experimental brain tumors. *J Neurooncol*, 2004. *68*(3): p. 225-32.

[91] Choti, M.A., et al., Intrahepatic FUdr delivered from biodegradable polymer in experimental liver metastases from colorectal carcinoma. *Proc of A.A.C.R.*, 1995. *36*: p. 309.

[92] Dang, W., et al., Covalent coupling of methotrexate to dextran enhances the penetration of cytotoxicity into a tissue-like matrix. *Cancer Res*, 1994. *54*(7): p. 1729-35.

[93] Sipos, E.P., et al., L-buthionine sulfoximine potentiates the antitumor effect of 4-hydroperoxycyclophosphamide when administered locally in a rat glioma model. *Neurosurgery*, 2001. *48*(2): p. 392-400.

[94] Hanes, J., et al., Controlled local delivery of interleukin-2 by biodegradable polymers protects animals from experimental brain tumors and liver tumors. *Pharm Res*, 2001. *18*(7): p. 899-906.

[95] Rhines, L.D., et al., Local immunotherapy with interleukin-2 delivered from biodegradable polymer microspheres combined with interstitial chemotherapy: a novel treatment for experimental malignant glioma. *Neurosurgery*, 2003. *52*(4872-9).

[96] Lesniak, M.S., J. Frazier, and H. Brem, Targeting Drugs to Tumors of the Central Nervous System. *Contemporary Cancer Research: Brain Tumors ed.* F. Ali-Osman, Humana Press Inc. Totowa, NJ, 2004.

[97] Lesniak, M.S. and H. Brem, Targeted therapy for brain tumours. *Nat Rev Drug Discov,* 2004. *3*(6): p. 499-508.

[98] Varallyay, P., et al., Comparison of two superparamagnetic viral-sized iron oxide particles ferumoxides and ferumoxtran-10 with a gadolinium chelate in imaging intracranial tumors. *Am J Neuroradiol*, 2002. *23*(4): p. 510-9.

[99] Brem, H. and R. Langer, Polymer-based drug delivery to the brain. *Sci Med*, 1996. *3*: p. 52-61.

In: Brain Cancer: Therapy and Surgical Interventions... ISBN 1-59454-974-5
Editor: Andrew V. Yang, pp. 23-44

Chapter II

Current Concepts and Experimental Strategies Concerning Local Drug Infusion Systems for Brainstem Tumors

R. J. Strege

Department of Neurosurgery, Klinikum Plau am See, Plau am See, Germany

B. S. Carson, Sr. and M. Guarnieri

The Johns Hopkins University School of Medicine, Baltimore, Maryland, USA

Abstract

Objective

Despite recent advances in surgical technology, many brain stem tumors, mainly diffuse pediatric gliomas, have been regarded as inoperable until today. Local drug delivery approaches to this eloquent area have therefore gained increasingly research interest. First experiments have been performed on rodents. This review describes the current experimental efforts and latest laboratory findings concerning local drug infusion systems for the brain stem.

Methods

The English-language literature on brain stem tumor models and therapy approaches for local drug delivery by infusion systems was reviewed using the MEDLINE Pub Med database (1966-present).

Results

Current concepts, drug delivery methods (high-flow and low-flow), animal models (rats, mice, monkeys), pharmacokinetic, radiologic and histologic data of drug distribution as well as clinical data of side effects such as neurotoxicity are presented.

Conclusion

Catheter implantation into the brainstem of animals for the purpose of drug delivery appears to be safely possible. On the basis of the currently available data, chronic drug delivery of certain agents seems to be tolerated in different animals in potentially effective doses. Clinico-neurological side effects are dose- and drug dependent and showed variability even in the same kind of animals. Local drug infusion systems will most likely become an important mechanism for drug delivery to the brainstem in the future. The preliminary findings have layed the groundwork for further investigations and give the hope for clinical trials in the future.

1. Introduction and Historical Background

Brainstem tumors of childhood have a poor prognosis. Approximately 300 new cases of brainstem gliomas are diagnosed yearly in the United States [71], about 70% of which are diffuse pontine gliomas [18]. The median survival of children with diffuse pontine gliomas is reported to be approximately 10 months [1], with 2-year survival rates of 10-15% [18, 76]. Neither chemotherapy nor radiation significantly prolongs the survival of these patients, according to the currently available data from trials with small numbers of patients from single institutions [21, 22, 52]. Low-grade lesions, that are rather rare, may, in contrast, respond to surgery, chemotherapy, and radiation, with 5-year survival rates of more than 50% [18, 76].

Since the prognosis for children with malignant brainstem tumors, i.e. diffuse (pontine) gliomas, appears to be mostly dismal, new therapeutic efforts must be evaluated. Systemic chemotherapy as well as all applied radiation modalities have uniformly failed. In addition, there have been significant side effects from systemic chemotherapy. Whereas radiation doses are limited to 5000-5500 rads [75] due to the danger of radiation necrosis in such an eloquent CNS area, systemic chemotherapies are limited by their systemic toxicity such as myelosuppression in particular because high concentrations of drug are necessary to cross the blood-brain barrier (BBB) and the blood-tumor barrier (BTB).

Research efforts have focused in recent years on local delivery of therapeutic agents to brainstem malignancies to overcome the limitations of systemic therapy. Diffuse pontine gliomas do not typically metastasize and are characterized by a relatively compact nature, a feature that seems ideal for effective local delivery strategies. Intratumoral (local) therapy increases tumor-drug ratios and decreases non-target side effects. Three main strategies for local therapy have evolved: (1) blood-brain-barrier disruption, (2) bolus injection, and (3) chronic infusions.

(1) RMP-7 is one of the prominent drug candidates that is able to transiently disrupt the BBB and hereby to enhance the efficacy of systemic therapy when given as co-infusion. There are, for example, several reports on phase 1 studies of carboplatin combined with RMP-7 which described acceptable safety in adults [12, 16, 19, 24, 57] and children [51, 71].

(2) Cytotoxic drugs have been locally injected into parenchyma or cerebrospinal fluid [8]. Despite high intratumoral drug doses, therapeutic effects were disappointing. First, it was supposed that intratumoral pressure may prevent diffusion of drugs throughout the tumor, so that only a small volume of tissue surrounding the drug source is treated [4, 32, 33, 47]. Second, it was recognized, that treatment-free periods after bolus injection allow recovery of the tumor and enrichment of drug-resistent tumor cells [3]. Third, tumors seemed to be not uniformly susceptible for brief drug exposure because of their microheterogeneity [31].

(3) It was hypothesized and proved to be valid in animal models that chronic delivery systems for intratumoral therapy overcome the relatively high tissue pressure in tumors and provide a prolonged interaction between tumor cells and drug [8]. Chronic delivery can be achieved in general by two different ways of drug application: chronic infusion by infusion pumps or by drug-releasing biodegradable polymers.

Both methods have been applied to supratentorial brain tumors. There is a large body of clinical and histologic evidence that convection-enhanced delivery can be safely applied in the cerebrum of rats [10, 25, 41, 56, 68], cats [4], primates [38, 54], and humans [30, 39, 53, 57, 67, 72]. Employment of easily implantable, osmotic mini pumps made chronic drug delivery to the brain possible. Nierenberg et al. [48]) intratumorally infused methotrexat into five patients with glioblastoma multiforme in 1991. Other drugs, that were given intratumorally, followed in subsequent clinical studies, such as paclitaxel, for example, very recently in 2004 [42].

Brem and coworkers [6] extensively investigated and established the implantation of biodegradable, drug-coated polymers into the wound cave after tumor resection. The working mechanisms of polymer-based infusion predominantly rely on diffusion. Carmustine (BCNU) was the first-generation drug and has become the standard therapy for recurrent glioblastoma multiforme. Its efficacy has been proved by several studies [6, 67]. Interstitial delivery of carboplatin via biodegradable polymers has been proved effective against experimental rat brain glioma: the best intracranial polymer dose was significantly more effective than the best systemic dose tested [50].

Until now, there have been, to our knowledge, no efforts to use infusion polymers to treat brainstem tumors, probably because such method seems to be less suitable for the treatment of inoperable malignancies. In contrast to infusion polymers, chronic infusion systems have been increasingly under investigation for the treatment of malignant brainstem tumors in recent years.

Kroin et al. [36] were the first who published experimental data on local delivery of cisplatin into the cerebellum of rats. Hereby, as early as 1982, they presented the proof of principle by their chronic low-flow infusion of cisplatin at flow rates of 0.9μl/h in a rat model. Furthermore, they infused in a clinical trial cisplatin for ten days at 0.5 μl/h into the cerebrum of a patient with recurrent malignant glioma and demonstrated the safety of infusion but without convincing efficacy in terms of survival [36]. That therapy approach was, however, not further followed mainly because of technical concerns about limited distribution capacity in relation to the often large tumor volume.

As a result from ongoing research in neurooncology, there has taken place something like a renaissance of local delivery approaches. In January 2003 a symposium was held to discuss the current state of progress and future challenges for the technique of convection enhanced delivery (CED) [69]. Therapeutic efforts for human glial tumors in general have over the past years been redirected towards a compartmental treatment concept [73]. Most recent development of numerous promising new drugs such as highly specific, targeted toxins [11], encouraged researchers to further investigate compartmental drug delivery strategies, even for brainstem regions.

2. Method of Literature Search and Results

The English-language literature on brain stem tumor models and therapy approaches for local drug delivery by infusion systems was reviewed using the MEDLINE Pub Med database (1966-present). We looked for the following search criteria: "brainstem infusions", "brainstem and local therapy", "brainstem and local infusion", "brainstem and local delivery", "brainstem and interstitial infusion", "convection-enhanced delivery", "brainstem tumor and animal model" and "brainstem and animal tumor model". There were found 741, 627, 215, 50, 12, 85, 3, and 105 listed papers, respectively.

Excluding all non topic-related papers such as reports on neurodegenerative diseases, for example, sixteen out of these papers contained experimental data on brainstem tumor models [34, 74], local infusion approaches to the brainstem [14, 28, 43, 45, 49, 60, 61, 63, 64, 65, 66] including the cerebellum [36], or both [9, 75]. Table 1 gives a survey on all sixteen papers. Despite some preliminary clinical trials on convection-enhanced delivery strategies in supratentorial tumors [30, 39], there have been, to our knowledge, no clinical trials of local infusion therapy for brainstem tumors conducted so far. All experimental data being available and presented here are therefore restricted to exclusively pre-clinical data.

3. Brainstem Tumor Models

Prior to investigate intratumoral drug treatments, development of experimental models of brainstem tumors was required. Apart from a few reports describing experimental models for cerebellar medulloblastoma (Schabet et al. [62] among others), there are, to our knowledge, only two animal tumor models for diffuse brainstem tumors, i.e. diffuse gliomas: the F 98 glioma and the 9 L gliosarcoma rodent cell line model. Both tumor models were primarily developed in supratentorial regions. The transfer of these tumor models from supratentorial cerebrum to brainstem was pioneered by the investigative group of Carson and coworkers [9, 74, 75] in the early years of the 21. century.

Table 1. A list of all published experimental data on brainstem tumor models and local infusion systems for brainstem tumor therapy

Experimental model			Parameters of infusion			Ref.
Animal	**Tumor**	**Infusate**	**Rate of infusion**	**Duration of infusion**	**Total volume of infusion**	
Fischer rats	F 98, 9 L	Carboplatin, dextrose	1 μl/h	chronic: 7d	~200μl	[9]
Fischer rat pups	F 98, 9 L	Tumor cells, saline	-	one time	2μl	[34]
Fischer rats	F 98	Carboplatin, dextrose	1μl/h	chronic :7d	~200μl	[75]
Fischer rats, Balb/C mice	F 98, 9 L EMT6,B16	Tumor cells, saline	0.5μl/min	one time	2μl	[74]
Fischer rats	((9 L))*	Carboplatin, Gemcitabine	0.5 μl/min	one time	40μl	[14]
Wistar rats	-	Cisplatin	0.9μl/h	chronic: 7d	~200μl	[36[
Sprague-Dawley rats	-	FITC-dextran, saline	7.9μl/h	chronic: 7d	1400μl	[49]
Sprague-Dawley rats	-	FITC-dextran, saline	0.1μl/min	one time	up to 4μl	[60]
Sprague-Dawley rats	-	FITC-dextran $\pm$ mannitol	0.1μl/min	one time	1μl	[61]
Sprague-Dawley rats	-	Carmustine	7.9μl/h	chronic: 1d	200μl	[63]
Sprague-Dawley rats	-	IL13-PE38QQR	7.9μl/h	chronic: 1d	200μl	[64]
Mice	-	Saline	0.25-8.0 μl/ h	chronic: 30d	up to 360μl	[28]
Cynomolgus monkeys	-	Carboplatin, saline	0.42μl/h	chronic: 90 d	900μl	[65]
Cynomolgus monkeys	-	Carboplatin	0.42μl/h	chronic: 30 d	300μl	[66]
Cynomolgus monkeys	-	Carboplatin	0.42μl/h	chronic: 29 d	292μl	[46]
Macaca monkeys	-	Gd-bound albumin	0.25-1μl/min	one time	85-120μl	[43]

* Tumor cell inoculation in frontal lobe only, not brainstem; "one time" means single short infusion

They established the successful implantation of $1x10^4$ [9, 74, 75] to $1x10^6$ cells [34] into the pontine rat brainstem according to the methods described for the first time by Wu et al. [74]. Microscopic examination of the tumor cell-challenged brains demonstrated that the tumors grew primarily at the site of the inoculation and spread along the path of the injection [74]. The histological appearance resembled cortical inoculations of the same tumor cell line with the exception of missing evidence of central necrosis at autopsy [74].

The inoculations produced reproducible survival curves with dose-dependent survival [74]. As expected, survival was significantly decreased in brainstem-challenged animals compared to similar tumor cell challenges in the parietal cortex. The median survival time of 14 days in Fischer rats inoculated with 10^4 9L cells into the brainstem, for example, was reproducibly shorter in contrast to 20 days when injections were made into the cortex [74]. The development of neurologic symptoms in tumor-challenged animals was consistent with mass effects of the tumor on centers of respiration and consciousness.

Most recently, Jallo et al. [34] successfully adapted the 9L and F98 tumor models to the neonatal brainstem by inoculating Fischer rat newborn pups (aged 12-24h) that were anesthetized by hypothermia with orthotopic tumor cells. Little or no morbidity was observed with injections of 3-3.5mm depth that ranged from the midline to approximately 1mm lateral [34]. Tumor growth was generally confined to the brainstem [34]. The maximum size of the tumors measured at autopsy was 4-5mm in diameter regardless of the number of cells injected [34].

In addition to the 9L and F98 tumor cell lines, the EMT6 breast tumor cell line and B16 melanoma cell line, that represent examples for the second and third most common intracranial CNS metastases, have been shown by Wu et al. [74] to be able to efficiently colonize the brainstem. They may serve as brainstem metastasis models in the future.

4. Interstitial Infusion Therapy into the Brainstem

4.1. Concepts and General Considerations

There are different terms in use, describing interstitial infusion. The most commonly used term may be *convection-enhanced delivery* that means delivery by *high-flow infusions* due to a pressure gradient. Its interstitial flux is based on bulk flow [4, 47] and largely independent of molecular weight (MW) and solutions are distributed in relatively homogeneous concentrations [17, 45, 59]. High-flow infusion at rates of 10-100μl/h can be differentiated from *low-flow infusion* at rates of 0.1-1μl/h that allows delivery due to a diffusion gradient. Bruce et al. [7] additionally used the term « intracerebral clysis" to describe convection-enhanced delivery in their studies on a frontal lobe rat glioma model. Kroin et al. [36] introduced additional terms such as chronic microinfusion or microperfusion. For the purpose of a nomenclature as uniform as possible, we prefer to use the terms "high-flow infusion" for infusion rates of $\geq$ 10 μl/h and "low-flow infusion" for infusion rates of $\leq$ 1μl/h in accordance with general literature data.

Pump-based interstitial infusion systems have been predominantly under investigation as alternative treatment protocols for inoperable brainstem tumors. Polymer-based infusion instead, which is mostly used as intracavitary approach after tumor resection, plays, to our knowledge, no (significant) role for delivery into the brainstem so far.

Whereas supratentorial cerebrum studies may focus on delivery into either gray or white matter, examination of delivery methods into pontine brainstem covers nearly exclusively white matter substance. That makes a difference concerning the size of infused molecules and the supposed main direction of infusate distribution. It was reported that convection-enhanced delivery infusions, i.e. high-flow infusions, follow isotropic white matter [26]. Furthermore, besides the parameters of infusion determining the infusate distribution, it depends upon the specific local environment which is more complex/dense in the brainstem and clearly distinct from the cerebrum. To serve as a potential alternative for therapeutic delivery in the treatment of diffuse pontine gliomas, the aim of all efforts must be to affect a large volume of the brainstem compartment.

4.2. Modality of Infusion

4.2.1. Site of Infusion and Injection Coordinates: Ventral versus Dorsal Route

Until now, dorsal routes have been clearly preferred and nearly exclusively used in research on brainstem infusion techniques (complete list of Table 1 and 2). Dorsal approaches have been considered to work generally well for inoculations [74], whereas ventral approaches seem to be more suitable for surgery in dogs, for example [35]. The commonly used approach has been the midline or paramedian dorsal approach to the examined animals. The placement of cannula was mostly performed by using a stereotactic frame, especially in rats. After the placement of cannula, tubing and osmotic mini pump have to be connected for chronic delivery. For this purpose, the mini pump is regularly implanted into a subcutaneous pocket of the neck for the duration of infusion.

Interaural, lateral, and depth coordinates have been as follows: *rats*: for pontine target: 2mm post lambdoid suture, 2mm lateral, 7 mm depht below dura [9, 73, 75], or 1mm post lambdoid suture, 1 to 2mm lateral, 3mm depth [34], or for pontine nucleus oralis (PnO): 1mm anterior to lambdoid suture, 1.4mm to the right of the sagittal suture, 7mm below dura [14, 49, 60, 61, 63, 64], or L-0, P-11, H-3 below the dura mater within the cerebellum [36]; *mize*: for pontine target: 1.5 to 2.5mm post lambdoid suture, 0 to 2mm lateral, 3.5mm depth [74]; and *monkeys*: for pontine target: 2.5cm below inion, 1.75mm anterior-posterior, -12.5 mm dorsoventral, 0mm mediolateral [46, 65, 66] or -6.0mm anterior-posterior, -12,5mm dorsoventral, 0mm mediolateral [43]. The coordinates for rats and mice were based on published stereotactic coordinates of mouse and rat anatomy, respectively [20, 54].

4.2.2. Size of Infusate Molecules: Macro- versus Micromolecular Substances

The delivery of macromolecules into the brainstem is of interest for two main reasons: first, many promising agents such as antibodies, gene vectors, and immunotoxins are macromolecules. Second, it is more difficult for macromolecules than micromolecules to pass the blood-brain-barrier. In addition, Mardor et al. [44] very recently found in a rat brain model that low-viscosity infusates tend to backflow along the catheter track whereas high-viscosity infusates tend to form efficient convection.

Micromolecular infusates into the brainstem comprised cisplatin (MW = 300kD), carboplatin (MW = 371kD), gemcitabine (MW = 300kD), and carmustine (MW = 214kD); macromolecular comprised FITC-dextran (MW = 20kD) and Gd-albumin (MW = 72kD)(see Table 1). The size limitation of particles that can be distributed with convection, i.e. high-flow-infusion, has not been established [10]. There is reported evidence that convection-enhanced infusion effectively distributes large molecules (MW 10 to 126kD) through grey matter [41]. Furthermore, it was shown that higher infusion rates are associated with greater backward leakage [10].

4.2.3. Rate of Infusion: High- versus Low-flow Infusion

High-flow infusions at rates of $\geq$ 10μl/h, that are often considered to be more potent than low-flow infusions, play a predominant role in brain regions other than the brainstem. Concerning the brainstem, in contrast, several researchers prefer low-flow infusions because of their less risk potential for brainstem damage. Bruce et al. [7], for example, stated that increased infusion rate into the brain caused increased intratumoral pressure.

4.2.4. Size and Consistency of Cannula: Flexible versus Rigid Catheter

Previous experiments for convective delivery to the cerebrum showed that increases in cannula diameter facilitate formation of a low-resistance pathway that follows the surface contours of the cannula [10]. In the most brainstem infusion experiments reported so far, nearly exclusively implantation of rigid catheters has been performed. Since most recently Guarnieri et al. [29], however, reported serious disadvantages of rigid compared to flexible catheters, such as unintended larger leak back flow along catheter, increasingly use of flexible catheters for brainstem infusion experiments can be expected for the future. The cannula diameter varied between different studies from 23 to 32 gauge cannulas.

5. Experiments and Limitations

5.1. Animal Models

As mentioned above (see section brainstem tumor models), there have been so far brainstem tumor models in Fischer rats only, such as F 98 glioma, 9 L gliosarcoma, EMT 6 breast tumor, and B16 melanoma. Published experiments on local delivery into the brainstem in neurooncological context have been conducted in rodents, i.e. some kinds of rats (such as Fischer, Wistar, and Sprague-Dawleys) and mice, and in primates, i.e. Cynomolgus as well as Macaca monkeys (Table 1). The studies can be divided into tumor establishing studies [34, 74], feasibility studies [14, 28, 36, 43, 46, 49, 60, 61, 63, 64, 65, 66] and only two efficacy studies comprising chronic delivery of carboplatin into the pontine brainstem in the F 98 and 9 L Fischer rat tumor model [9, 75].

5.2. Infused Substances/Infusates

Carboplatin represents the most often examined drug for local delivery into the brainstem in general and into brainstem tumor tissue in particular. It was chosen for the respective studies due to several reasons as explained by Carson et al. [9]: the drug is widely used in laboratory research and clinical neurooncology for primary and secondary lesions including pediatric brainstem tumors [12, 15, 16, 19, 23, 24, 27, 50, 51, 52, 55, 71], it is relatively stable in dextrose solutions at 37°, and tissue distributions can be estimated by atomic absorption spectroscopy.

Likewise, gemcitabine was selected together with carboplatin because both drugs are water-soluble so that they are sequestered on whichever side of the blood-brain-barrier they are placed [14]. Carmustine is the first and best examined drug for polymer-based infusion systems [6, 40, 67]. The glioma specific, chimeric cytotoxin IL13-PE38QQR was chosen as candidate therapeutic agent that has been already tested in clinical studies for recurrent supratentorial malignant gliomas in adults [40, 53, 57]. Gd-bound albumin [43] and FITC-dextran [49, 60, 61] were selected as model macromolecular solutes because of their imaging-suited characteristics.

Table 2 summarizes experimental designs of combinations categorized according to variables such as type of infusate, animal, presence of a tumor, and duration of infusion. The type of infusate could be further subdivided into four substance classes: (a) tumor cells, (b) saline, (c) visible marker solutes such as FITC-dextran and Gd-bound-albumin or (d) therapeutic cytotoxic drugs such as carboplatin, cisplatin, gemcitabine, carmustine and IL13-PE38QQR as immunotoxin-based drug. Nine different combinations of infusate + animal + duration of infusion ± tumor could be classified at all.

Table 2. *S*ystematically listed experimental combinations for local brainstem infusion

Type of main infusate	Animal tumor	Infusion duration	Clinical toxicity	Histology	Distribution monitoring	Ref.
Tumor cells, saline	Rats/ F 98,) L	one time	-	+	MRI [73]	[34, 73]
Saline	Mice/ -	chronic	+	-	-	[28]
FITC-dextran	Rats/ -	one time	-	+	fluorescence	[60, 61]
FITC-dextran	Rats/ -	chronic	-	+	fluorescence	[49]
Gd-bound albumin	Monkeys/-	one time	-	+	MRI	[43]
Carboplatin, gemcitabine	Rats/-	one time	-	+	-	[14]
Cisplatin, IL13, Carmustine	Rats/-	chronic	-	+ [63, 64]	AAS [36]	[36, 63, 64]
Carboplatin	Monkeys/-	chronic	+	+ [65]	AAS, MRI* [65, 66]	[46, 65, 66]
Carboplatin, Doxorubicin	Rats/ F 98, 9 L	chronic	+	+	AAS, MRI*	[9, 75]

FITC: fluorescein isothiocyanate; Gd: gadolinium; AAS: atomic absorption spectroscopy; MRI: magnetic resonance imaging; MRI*: MRI monitoring for toxicity, not for direct drug delivery extent

5.3. Parameters of Infusion

The rate of infusion varied in one time delivery between 0.1 and 1 µl/min. The rate of infusion in chronic delivery studies comprised flow rates of about 1 µl/h [9, 36, 75] or 7.9µl/h [49, 63, 64] in rats, 0.25-8.0µl/h in mice [28] and 0.42µl/h in monkeys [46, 65, 66]. The flow rates of 7.9µl/h were nearer to high-flow than low-flow infusion rates according to definitions as described above. The duration of chronic infusions varied from one day (= 24 hours) to 90 days, with a main duration of 7 days in rats [9, 36, 49, 75] and about 30 days in monkeys [46, 66].

The total volume of infusion ranged in the group of one time delivery from 1 to 120µl and in the goup of chronic delivery from 200 to 1400µl, respectively.

5.4. Feasibility

All studies listed in Table 1 and 2 proved the principal feasibility of both one time and chronic local delivery of infusates to the pontine brainstem. Initial studies focussed on safety of inserting a cannula into the pontine brainstem of animals and infusing nontherapeutic agents. Subsequent studies focussed on the chronic delivery of therapeutic agents. Procedural-related technical problems were mainly associated with the cannula system in terms of unintended leak back flow along the path of cannula/catheter into the subdural space.

Using rigid catheters resulted in partly unexpected, i.e. unreliable, drug distribution patterns. The expected approximately bell-shaped curve with a maximum drug concentration near the infusion point and approximately equal, declining concentrations rostral and caudal to the infusion could be observed in only about half of the rats examined by Guarnieri et al. [29]: replacement of rigid infusion tubes with flexible tubing significantly increased the reliability of local CNS drug infusions into the cerebrum.

5.5. Safety and Toxicity

5.5.1. Clinical Effects: Toxicity

One time midline injections of 2 µl saline and injections 1mm and up to 2mm to either side of the midline through the cerebellum and fouth ventricle were tolerated without neurologic symptoms or mortality in mice and rats [74]. Significant morbidity was, however, apparent in the immediate postoperative period when the following interaural, lateral and depth coordinates (mm) were used for injections in mice: -2.5/3.5/3.5 and -2.5/2.0/5.5 and in rats: -2.0/-5.0/7.0 and -2/-2/9.0 [74]. Such mice did not revive from anesthesia and showed shallow or irregular respiration followed by death within 8 hours, whereas rats did revive but were lethargic and failed to drink or eat [74].

These results reflect the sensitivity of the brainstem to injections outside safe coordinates. In addition, Jallo et al. [34] observed in their neonatal rat model little or no morbidity with 2µl injections of saline or tumor cell suspensions that ranged from the midline to approximately 1mm lateral. In this model it has to be taken into account that 5 to 21% of animal pups were removed by their mothers after getting injections and that increasing skills of the examiner in terms of a learning curve significantly decreased the percentage of pup rejection by the mother [34].

Guarnieri et al. [28] presented experimental data that morbidity and mortality rates increased with increasing chronic flow rates of saline into the brainstem of mice and rats:

mouse survival on day 2 was 2/3, 1/3 and 0/3 for flow rates of 0.25µl/h, 1µl/h and 8µl/h, respectively. Several researchers observed neither neurological deficits occuring after one time delivery nor chronic delivery of FITC-dextran at a flow rate of 7.9µl/h into the pontine rat brainstem [49, 60, 61]. All studies using FITC-dextran for brainstem infusion have consistently demonstrated that chronic nearly high-flow infusion did not result in any clinical deterioration, raised intracranial pressure -as far as examined - , or histological evidence of disrupted cytoarchitecture other than that at the site of cannula insertion. But Bruce et al. [7] found increased intratumoral pressures with increased flow rates into the brain.

In contrast to that data, experiments of Carson et al. [9] gave evidence that mortality of rats chronically infused with saline was higher the higher the flow rate was. To investigate the feasibility of local therapy, they infused rat brainstems at 0.25-10µl/h for one or more days. Hereby, chronic infusion rates of approximately 2.5µl/h were generally tolerated. Chronic flow rates of 5-10µl/h, however, which are acceptable in the brain, were partly traumatic for the brainstem: None of the 5 rats infused at 10µl/h survived to day 14 and three of 10 rats infused at 5µl/h died by day 14 [9].

Lonser et al. [43] infused the brainstem of three Macaca mulatta monkeys with 85, 110 and 120µl volumes of Gd-bound albumin, respectively, at single, short flow rates of 0.25 to 1µl/min without any signs of neurological deficits in the 35 days-follow up period. Since then, safe single infusions of a short duration of nontherapeutic agents have been documented in the brainstem of rats [34, 60, 61, 74], mice [74], and monkeys [43]. Concerning chronic infusions of nontherapeutic agents, however, flow-rate dependent toxicity was reported in some rat and mouse studies, as mentioned above [9,28].

Few studies have addressed the concerns regarding the potential toxicity of locally administered therapeutic agents. Local delivery of carboplatin and gemcitabine at constant flow rates of 0.5µl/h and 80min duration [14], carmustin and IL-13 at flow rates of 7.9µl/h and 24h duration [63, 64] as well as cisplatin at a flow rate of 0.9µl/h for seven days into the rat brainstem (Kroin, 1982) have all been reported without occurence of any clinical toxicity in the respective animals. Chronic delivery ($\geq$ 7 days) of carboplatin, however, showed both, dose-escalating toxicity in rats and monkeys [46, 65, 66, 75].

Local delivery of carboplatin predominantly caused localized neurotoxicity [46, 65, 66, 75]: Wu et al. [75] determined in their rat brainstem tumor model study that the maximally tolerated dose (MTD) of carboplatin delivered into the rat brainstem was a concentration of 0.5mg/ml at a flow rate of 1.0µl/h for 7 days. The animals receiving a pump loaded with either 2.0mg/ml or 4.0mg/ml of carboplatin showed unacceptable toxicity with either 60% (3/5) or 80% (4/5) of the animals dying before day 10, respectively. A concentration of 1.0mg/ml of carboplatin showed some toxicity with an animal dying on day 11.

Storm et al. [65] initially infused the brainstem of two primates with saline at a constant flow-rate of 0.42µl/h for 90 days without signs of neurological deficits or changes in grooming, habits, appetite, or activity. A third animal receiving 0.1xMTD = approximately 0.25mg/kg of carboplatin at the same constant flow-rate remained unremarkable. Two other primates receiving 1xMTD showed first behavioural changes when the delivered dose of carboplatin reached 486 and 590µg, respectively. In conclusion, continuous infusions exceeding 400µg of carboplatin lead to neurotoxicity in 3-8kg nonhuman primates and infusions exceeding 180µg in 4 days produced rapidly progressive toxicity [65].

Likewise, Strege et al. [66] reported dose-dependent neurotoxicity in terms of particularly ataxia, abnormal gaze, and lethargy in chronically-infused Cynomolgus monkeys. The clinical course of monkeys receiving 0.1xMTD of carboplatin was unremarkable for the complete time period of 4-5 weeks of infusion [66]. Animals of the 0.3xMTD and 1xMTD group showed slow movement and ataxia from around day 30 on, corresponding to 240-276 and 590-694µg total dose of carboplatin, respectively. Animals of the 3xMTD group displayed rapidly progressing ataxia and lethargy already within day 4-10. In addition, it was assumed that nausea may have been a side effect because a majority of animals lost weight during the infusions [66].

Significant infusion-related systemic side effects such as pathological blood cell changes were not observed [65, 66]. The transient drop in the eosinophil count recorded in the steroid-free animals in the 1xMTD group might have been indicated hypersensitivity reactions that have been previously reported in association with carboplatin infusions [77].

May et al. [46] examined three monkeys weighing 4 to 6 kg and receiving a total infused dosage of 694µg carboplatin (approximately 0.25 mg/kg = estimated maximum tolerated dose (MTD) for a 3 kg monkey). They found, as recorded by evoked auditory potentials, increased hearing tresholds of about 10 dB 1 year after drug treatment. This hearing loss was modest in comparison to that previously observed under systemic carboplatin infusion, but statistically significant ($p < 0.05$).

The comparison and interpretation of the different studies has to be limited due to large heterogeneity of experimental designs in general and infusion parameters in particular. Nevertheless, some tendentious conclusions can be drawn. Conclusively, there is a drug and dose- as well as flow-dependent localized toxicity that has to be specifically defined for each experimental setting itself. The preliminary data suggest that systemic side effects, in contrast, do not play a significant role in both one time and chronic local delivery into the brainstem.

5.5.2. Clinical Effects: Efficacy

There are two efficacy studies conducted in tumor-bearing and carboplatin-infused rats which have been addressed to examine survival data [9, 75]. Carson et al. [9] examined Fischer 344 rats in which five days after tumor inoculations, 0.5mg/ml solutions of carboplatin were infused at 1µl/h for 7 days. Compared to control groups that survived 13-17 days with F98 tumors and 22-23 days with 9L tumors, animals locally infused with 0.1mg of carboplatin survived 27-30 days ($p > 0.0003$). Likewise, Wu et al. [75] reported similar findings: carboplatin delivered locally by the 7-day 200µl-1.0 µl/h Alzet osmotic pump significantly prolonged survival in the F98 glioma brainstem tumor model. Control rats receiving dextrose had a median survival of 14 days (range 9~20), whereas animals receiving 0.5mg/ml carboplatin had a median survival of 36.5 days (range 19~54 days; $p < 0001$) Notably, no survival advantage was observed in a group that received a systemic injection of 30mg/kg carboplatin alone (median survival, 15 days, range 10~21 days). The clinical efficacy in both studies corresponded to the drug distribution measured by the atomic absorption sprectroscopy as platinum surrogate assay (see below).

5.5.3. Histological Effects

Apart from two exclusive studies on establishing of brainstem tumor models, there are eleven study reports providing data of histopathological findings after local brainstem infusion by FITC-dextran [49, 60, 61] or Gd-bound albumin [43] as model/marker solutes, or therapeutic drugs [9, 14, 43, 63, 64, 65, 75]. Histopathological analysis by standard H&E staining and partly additional staining methods uniformly yielded some (minor) pathological tissue changes around the catheter tip/cannula track. This counts equally for tissue infused by therapeutic infusates as well as non-therapeutic agents. These pathological findings were consistently interpreted as clinically no significant. They included small amounts of gliosis, tissue disruption, microhaematomas, and inflammatory/pleomorphic cells.

Notably, Occhiogrosso et al. [49] observed after seven days of delivery cavitary lesions along the cannula track, ranging in size from 400μm to 0.32cm, that were mostly associated with inflammatory cells and with bacteria (cocci) in two cases. Additional changes associated with the lesions included swollen axons, hemosiederin-laden macrophages, astrocytosis, microgliosis, and collections of plasma cells [49]. The animals showed no clinical deficits so that the significance of such findings for human trials remains unclear.

While carboplatin delivered to rat brainstem at single flow rates of 0.5μl/min did not cause any apparent tissue changes beyond the area of catheter tip/cannula track [14], dose-dependently increasing areas of tissue damage such as necrosis were observed in chronically carboplatin-infused (0.42μl/h) primates [65]. The focus of necrosis was rostral to the tissue section containing the maximum tissue concentration of platinum. The area of necrosis in animals receiving 0.25mg/kg carboplatin (= 1xMTD) reached approximately 5mm in diameter and was coincident with the hyperintense signal and enhancement observed by MRI. In correspondence to survival effects in tumor model experiments, tumor tissue of F98 challenged rats showed a significant positively stained section for apoptosis and extensive necrosis compared to control animals [9, 75].

5.6. Distribution of Infusate and Monitoring of Distribution

Few reports contain data about distribution analysis of nontherapeutic agents locally delivered to normal pontine brainstem, i.e. FITC-dextran in rats [49, 60, 61] and GD-bound albumin in monkeys [43]. The volume of distribution (Vd) increased linearly along with the volume of infusion (Vi) of Gd-bound albumin [43] as well as FITC-dextran [60, 61]. The concentration across the perfused region was homogeneous, as assessed by cross-sectional line profiles [43]. The Vd/Vi ratio over the volumes infused with Gd-bound albumin was 8.7±1.2 (mean±SD)(Lonser). Substantially larger Vd/Vi ratios (mean 14-30.9) were found by Sandberg et al. [60] who examined local delivery of FITC-dextran at a constant rate (0.1μl/min) into the rat pontine nucleus oralis (PnO) until volumes of 0.5, 1, 2 and 4μl were reached. The volumes of distribution were not significantly increased by co-infusion of mannitol in experiments where 1μl of FITC-dextran was administered at a constant rate (0.1μl/min). Last, Occhiogrosso et al. [49] reported Vd/Vi ratios of 65.3-124.7 (mean) after infusates of 200μlVi for 24h and 2ml for 7 days at a flow rate of 7.9μl/h.

The higher Vd/Vi ratio of similar substances in the brainstem than that in gray [10] or white matter [4] in previous studies may indicate that the interstitial space of the brainstem is small compared with these other regions of the CNS because distribution is inversely related to the size of the extracellar space of the infused region [43]: Proportionally lesser interstitial space due to densely packed white matter tracts appears to permit rapid filling of clinically relevant portions of tissue [43].

In studies examining chronic delivery of carboplatin [9, 65] or cisplatin [36], platinum levels were assayed using an atomic absorption spectrophotometer to estimate the distribution of infused carboplatin or cisplatin, respectively. The distribution of carboplatin seen in normal brainstem of primates [65] was similar to reported values for carboplatin distribution in rodent brainstem with or without tumor [9] and cisplatin in rodent cortex and cerebellum [36]. After one week of low-flow infusion, the drug uniformly showed a symmetrical volume of distribution approximately 1 cm in diameter. The maximum tissue concentration was found near the infusion site, partly more rostral, partly more caudal.

Platinum levels greater than 10μg/g of tissue 8mm rostral and 4mm caudal to the infusion cannulas in the carboplatin study of Carson et al. [9] and platinum tissue levels of 2ng/mg over 1-cm region of brain in the cisplatin study of Kroin et al. [36] suggested that infusions distributed pharmacologically relevant levels through a volume of tissue of at least 0.5cm in diameter. The drug distribution profile of low-flow brainstem infusions such as carboplatin was characterized by steep concentration gradients and limited area of distribution compared to (near) high-flow infusions as FITC-dextran. This difference of high flow and low-flow infusion has been already previously described in cerebrum studies [41]. Furthermore, Liebermann et al. [41] stated that bulk flow penetration is limited only by the maximum allowable pumping pressure to the distance where spherical spread of the infusate has reduced the bulk flow velocity and corresponding flux to that characteristic of diffusion: radial distances generally on the order of 1.5cm, corresponding to the volumes of $14cm^3$ [41].

Most interestingly, modifying variables such as dose, volume and flow rate of infusion, Kroll et al. [37] concluded from their results that dose rather than convection (high-flow) might be the most important variable in volume of distribution. This observation contrasts with the findings of Chen et al. [10] who used convection to deliver 4μl of ^4C albumin to the striatum of 40 rats. They reported that the rate of infusion and cannula size can significantly affect convective distribution of molecules whereas variations in infusate concentrations have no effect in their animal model.

Imaging methods for distribution analysis, that have been mentioned above, represent surrogate assays only. The use of a fluorescence-labeled infusate prevents any qualitative and quantitative assessment [43, 60, 61]. In cases of carboplatin delivery, measurement of platinum levels by atomic absorption spectroscopy (AAS) enables only to detect platinum levels $\geq$ 2μg/l. Finally, MR-measured volumes of distribution may differ from tissue volume of distribution as measured by histochemical staining. Kroll et al. [36], for example, who examined the distribution of monocrystalline iron oxide nanocompounds in vivo by MR and by staining for iron.

Conclusively, differences in methodology make comparison between various studies quite difficult. Indirect monitoring of drug delivery extent can be achieved by the above mentioned methods representing surrogate assays. Other imaging methods that were primarily used in brain studies for the monitoring of toxicity have been SPECT [39] and diffusion MRI [13].

5.7. Interaction with other Active Substances Such as Mannitol and Steroids

Sandberg et al. [61] concluded from their experimental results that – in contrast to their expectations - neither systemic administration nor co-infusion of hyperosmolar mannitol significantly affects distribution parameters for convection-enhanced delivery of FITC-dextran. Similarly, they observed that mannitol administration by either means failed to significantly alter maximal cross-sectional area of fluorescence or cranio-caudal extent of fluorescence [61].

Strege et al. [66] reported that dexamethasone-treated primates displayed signs of neurotoxicity earlier and of a different type than non dexamethasone-treated animals that have been chronically infused with similar doses of carboplatin at the same constant flow rate of 0.42μl/h: these animals developed a vacant stare before occuring ataxia in week 4. They concluded that prophylactic steroids, 1mg/kg/day oral dexamethasone, appeared to have no protective effect on the development of clinical and radiographic signs in monkeys treated at 1xMTD levels of carboplatin.

6. Conclusions and Perspectives

The preliminary preclinical studies that have been conducted so far gave evidence for the feasibility and efficacy of local brainstem infusions of pump-delivered micro- and macromolecular solutes. Local delivery of carboplatin as the best examined candidate drug can be performed in efficient and stable doses with tolerable toxicity for at least 28 days. Systemic side effects of infusion were nearly not apparent in any examined infusate. Local toxicity corresponded to histopathological changes and showed both dose- and flow rate-dependency. Pharmacologically active concentrations of carboplatin were achieved by chronic infusion at a low-flow rate over a pontine tissue area of about 1 cm in diameter in tumor- as well as non tumor-bearing animals. Rat brainstem infusions at high(er) flow rates may lead to greater volumes of distribution but also enhance the risk for associated clinical morbidity and mortality as well as histopathological damage of unknown significance yet.

The preliminary experimental data suggest that currently caution is indicated concerning high-flow infusions for the brainstem. General conclusions from the present studies are somewhat limited by their small number, heterogeneity, by limited ability of direct measurement of infusate distribution and tissue effects and by the lack of a sufficiently representative animal model. To date, there is still not any good representative model of diffuse pontine gliomas. No currently available tumor model simulates exactly the unique features of diffuse pontine gliomas such as in particular the infiltrative nature and expansion along white matter tracts.

F 98 and 9 L tumors in the pontine brainstem of rodents such as rats and mice represent the best models we have today. As the next step, nonhuman primate models for brainstem tumors are required to sufficiently bridge the gap between rodent studies and safety studies in humans, because only non-tumor nonhuman primate models have been developed so far. An ideal delivery model would allow for the successful distribution of large-molecular-weight substances in a safe, reliable, and homogeneous manner over large anatomical volumes that could be monitored in vivo by using conventional noninvasive imaging methods [43].

The distribution profile of a certain drug not only depends upon the features of target tissue, size and concentration of that drug, but also upon additional properties such as the kind of receptor binding. Distribution patterns therefore have to be determined for each drug and its target region separately. Our understanding of the pharmacokinetics behind this form of drug delivery is just in developmental stages and better mathematical models are needed to correctly characterize such distribution patterns. The present work and preliminary findings, however, greatly encourage future efforts for local delivery strategies and strengthen the compartmental treatment concept for diffuse pontine gliomas. All what we know today about the biological behaviour of gliomas, increasingly call for a compartmental therapy with the aim not only to treat visible tumor-infiltrated tissue but to treat also the tissue that is not visibly infiltrated by the tumor.

Several researchers argue to start clinical trials for local delivery now [28] because of the dismal prognosis of such a disease. Currently, low-flow infusion systems seem to be more preferable than high-flow ones due to less risk potential. The disadvantage of lower distribution volumes in terms of limited efficacy may be compensated by several possible strategies that may be employed in the future. These may include testing various locations for catheter placement, inserting multiple catheters, using drug combinations or using new, more specific and potent drugs. It can be speculated that new gene vectors or immunotherapy agents in the future may potentially provide greater efficacy than previous conventional drugs. Both gene therapy and immunotherapy showed at least promising potential in preclinical experiments although gene therapy has not been clinically successful up to now.

Nevertheless, ongoing laboratory research is strongly mandatory including development of better animal models, optimization of infusion parameters, analysis of infusate distribution and effects, and designs of new drugs. Innovative imaging methods can be certainly expected for the next future that will further facilitate this work. In addition, electrophysiological monitoring such as somatosensory evoked potentials and/or brainstem evoked potentials may make procedures such as cannula placement as well as interstitial drug infusion safer in the future.

References

[1] Abbott R, Goh KYC. Brainstem gliomas. In: Albright L, Pollack I, Adelson, D, editors. *Principles and Practices of Pediatric Neurosurgery.* New York: Thieme Medical Publishers; 1999; pp 629-640.

[2] Bakhshi, S; North, RB. Implantable pumps for drug delivery to the brain. *J Neuro-Oncol* (1995) 26: 133-139.

[3] Bailar, JC 3rd; Gornik, HL. Cancer undefeated. *N Engl J Med* (1997) 336: 1569-1574.

[4] Bobo, RH; Laske, DW; Akbasak, A; Morrison, PF; Dedrick, RL; Oldfield, EH. Convection-enhanced delivery of macromolecules in the brain. *Proc Natl Acad Sci USA* (1994) 91: 2076-2080.

[5] Bouvier, G; Penn, RD; Kroin, JS; Beique, R; Guerard, MJ. Direct delivery of medication into a brain tumor through multiple chronically implanted catheters. *Neurosurgery* (1987) 20: 286-291.

[6] Brem, H; Pfantadosi, S; Purger, PC; Walker, M; Selker, R; Vick, NA; Black, K; Sisti, M; Brem, S; Mohr, G; et al. Placebo-controlled trial of safety and efficacy of intraoperative controlled delivery by biodegradable polymers of chemotherapy for recurrent gliomas. *Lancet* (1995) 345: 1008-1012.

[7] Bruce, JN; Falavigna, A; Johnson, JP; Hall, JS; Birch, BD; Yoon, JT; Wu, EX; Fine, RL; Parsa, AT. Intracerebral clysis in a rat glioma model. *Neurosurgery* (2000) 46: 683-91.

[8] Carson, BS Sr; Guarnieri, M. Local therapy for brain tumors. *Adv Clin Neurosci* (2002) 12: 89-99.

[9] Carson, BS; Wu, QZ; Tyler, B; Sukay, L; Raychaudhuri, R; DiMeco, F; Clatterbuck, R; Olivi, A; Guarnieri, M. New approach to tumor therapy for inoperable areas of the brain: chronic intraparenchymal drug delivery. *J Neurooncol* (2002) 60: 151-158.

[10] Chen, MY; Lonser, RR; Morrison, PF; Governale, LS; Oldfield, EH. Variables affecting convection-enhanced delivery to the striatum: a systemic examination of rate of infusion, cannula size, infusate concentration, and tissue-cannula sealing time. *J Neurosurg* (1999) 90: 315-320.

[11] Chiocca, EA; Broaddus, WC; Gillies, GT; Visted, T; Lamfers, ML. Neurosurgical delivery of chemotherapeutics, targeted toxins, genetic and viral therapies in neuro-oncology. *J Neuro-Oncol* (2004) 69: 101-117.

[12] Cloughesy, TF; Black, KL; Gobin, YP; Farahani, K; Nelson, G; Villablanca, P; Kabbinavar, F; Vineula, F; Wortel, CH. Intra-arterial Cereport (RMP-7) and carboplatin: a dose escalation study for recurrent malignant gliomas. *Neurosurgery* (1999) 44: 270-278.

[13] Croteau, D; Walbridge, S; Morrison, PF; Butman, JA; Vortmeyer, AO; Johnson, D; Oldfield, EH; Lonser, RR. Real-time in vivo imaging of the convective distribution of a low-molecular-weight tracer. *J Neurosurg* (2005) 102: 90-97.

[14] Degen, JW; Walbridge, S; Vortmeyer, AO; Oldfield, EH; Lonser, RR. Safety and efficacy of convection-enhanced delivery of gemcitabine or carboplatin in a malignant glioma model in rats. *J Neurosurg* (2003) 99: 893-898.

[15] Dunkel, IJ; Boyett, JM; Yates, A; Rosenblum, M; Garvin, JH Jr; Bostrom, BC; Goldman, S; Sender, LS; Gardner, SL; Li, H; Allen, JC; Finlay, JL. Children's Cancer Group. High-dose carboplatin, thiotepa, and etoposide with autologus stem-cell rescue for patients with recurrent medulloblastoma. *J Clin Oncol* (1998) 16: 222-228.

[16] Emerich, DF; Winn, SR; Snodgrass, P; LaFreniere, D; Agostino, M; Wiens, T; Xiong, H; Bartus, RT. Injectable chemotherapeutic microspheres and glioma II: enhanced survival following implantation into deep inoperable tumors. *Pharm Res* (2000) 17: 1212-1219.

[17] Fenstermacher, JD; Kaye, T. Drug "diffusion" within the brain. *Ann NY Acad Sci* (1988) 531: 29-39.

[18] Fisher, PG; Breiter, SN; Carson, BS; Wharam, MD; Williams, JA; Weingart, JD; Foer, DR; Goldthwaite, PT; Tihan, T; Burger, PC. A clinicopathologic reappraisal of brain

stem tumor classification: identification of pilocytic astrocytoma and fibrillary astrocytoma as distinct entities. *Cancer* (2000) 89: 1569-1576.

[19] Ford, J; Osborn, C; Barton, T; Bleehen, NM. A phase I study of intravenous RMP-7 with carboplatin in patients with progression of malignant glioma. *Eur J Cancer* (1998) 34: 1807-1811.

[20] Franklin, KBJ; Paxinos, G. The mouse brain in stereotaxic coordinates. *Academic Press*, San Diego, CA, 1997.

[21] Freeman, CR. Hyperfractionated radiotherapy for diffuse intrinsic brain stem tumors in children. *Pediatr Neurosurg* (1996) 24: 103-110.

[22] Freeman, CR; Perilongo, G. Chemotherapy for brain stem gliomas. *Childs Nerv Syst* (1999) 15: 545-553.

[23] Friedman, HS; Lovell, S; Rasheed, K; Friedman, AH. Treatment of adults with progressive oligodendroglioma with carboplatin. *Med Pediatr Oncology* (1998) 31: 16-18.

[24] Gregor, A; Lind, M; Newman, H; Grant, R; Hadley, DM; Barton, T; Osborn, C. Phase II studies of RMP-7 and carboplatin in the treatment of recurrent high grade glioma. RMP-7 European Study Group. *J Neurooncol* (1999) 44: 137-145.

[25] Groothuis, DR; Ward, S; Itskovich, AC; Dobrescu, C; Allen, CV; Dills, C; Levy, RM. Comparison of ^{14}C-sucrose delivery to the brain by intravenous, intraventricular, and convection-enhanced intracerebral infusion. *J Neurosurg* (1999) 90: 321-331.

[26] Groothuis, DR. The blood-brain and blood-tumor barriers: a review of strategies for increasing drug delivery. *Neuro-Oncology* (2000) 2: 45-59.

[27] Gruber, ML; Glass, J; Choudhri, H; Nirenberg, A. Carboplatin chemotherapy before irradiation in newly diagnosed glioblastoma multiforme. *Am J Clin Oncol* (1998) 21: 338-340.

[28] Guarnieri, M; Carson, BS. Chronic local therapy for brainstem tumors. (letter) *Neurosurgery* (2004) 54: 1025-1026.

[29] Guarnieri, M; Carson, BS; Khan, A; Penno, M; Jallo, GI. Flexible versus rigid catheters for chronic administration of exogenous agents into central nervous system tissues. *J Neurosci Methods* (2005) 144: 147-152.

[30] Hall, WA; Rustamzadeh, E; Asher, AL. Convection-enhanced delivery in clinical trials. *Neurosurg Focus* (2003) 14: e2.

[31] Haroun, RI; Brem, H. Local drug delivery. *Current Opinions in Oncology* (2000) 12: 1887-1893.

[32] Jain, RK. Barriers to drug delivery in solid tumors. *Scientific American* (1994) 271: 58-65.

[33] Jain, RK. Delivery of molecular medicine to solid tumors. *Science* (1996) 271: 1079-1080.

[34] Jallo, GI; Penno, M; Sukay, L; Liu, JY; Tyler, B; Lee, J; Carson, BS; Guarnieri , M. Experimental models of brainstem tumors: development of a neonatal rat model. *Childs Nerv Syst* (2005) 21: 399-403.

[35] Klopp, LS; Simpson, ST; Sorjonen, DC; Lenz, SD. Ventral surgical approach to the caudal brain stem in dogs. *Vet Surg* (2000) 29: 533-542.

[36] Kroin, JS; Penn, RD. Intracerebral chemotherapy: chronic microinfusion of cisplatin. *Neurosurgery* (1982) 10: 349-354.

[37] Kroll, RA; Pagel, MA; Muldoon, LL; Roman-Goldstein, S; Neuwelt, EA. Increasing volume of distribution to the brain with interstitial infusion: dose, rather than convection, might be the most important factor. *Neurosurgery* (1996) 38: 746-754.

[38] Laske, DW; Morrison, PF; Lieberman, DM, Corthesy, ME; Reynolds, JC; Stewart-Henney, PA, Koong, SS; Cummins, A; Paik, CH, Oldfield, EH. Chronic interstitial infusion of protein to primate brain: determination of drug distribution and clearance with single-photon emission computerized tomography imaging. *J Neurosurg* (1997) 87: 586-594.

[39] Laske, DW; Youle, RJ, Oldfield, EH. Tumor regression with regional distribution of the targeted toxin TF-CRM107 in patients with malignant brain tumors. *Nat Med* (1997) 3: 1362-1368.

[40] Lawrence, KF; Ewend, MG; Sills, A; Sipos, EP; Thompson, R; Watts, M; Colvin, OM; Brem, H; Saltzman, WM. Pharmacokinetics of interstitial delivery of carmustine, 4-hydroperoxycyclophosphamide, and paclitaxel from a biodegradable polymer implant in the monkey brain. *Cancer Res* (1998) 58: 672-684.

[41] Lieberman, DM, Laske, DW; Morrison, PF; Bankiewicz, KS; Oldfield, EH. Convection-enhanced distribution of large molecules in gray matter during interstitial drug infusion. *J Neurosurg* (1995) 82: 1021-1029.

[42] Lidar, Z; Mardor, Y; Jonas, T; Pfeffer, R; Faibel, M; Nass, D; Hadani, M; Ram, Z. Convection-enhanced delivery of paclitaxel for the treatment of recurrent malignant glioma: a phase I/II clinical study. *J Neurosurg* (2004) 100: 472-479.

[43] Lonser, RR; Walbridge, S; Garmestani, K; Butman, JA, Walters, HA, Vortmeyer, AO, Morrison, PF; Brechbiel, MW; Oldfield, EH. Succesful and safe perfusion of the primate brainstem: in vivo magnetic resonance imaging of macromolecular distribution during infusion. *J Neurosurg* (2002) 97: 905-913.

[44] Mardor, Y; Rahav, O; Zauberman, Y; Lidar, Z; Ocherashvilli, A; Daniels, D; Roth, Y, Maier, SE; Orenstein, A, Ram, Z. Convection-enhanced drug delivery: increased efficacy and magnetic resonance image monitoring. *Cancer Res* (2005) 65: 6858-63.

[45] Marmarou, A; Nakamura, T; Tanaka, K. The kinetics of fluid movement through brain tissue. *Semin Neurol 4* (1984) 4: 439-444.

[46] May, BJ; Guarnieri, M; Carson, BS; Bachani, A; Jallo, GI. Long-term effects of carboplatin brainstem infusions on hearing tresholds in monkeys. *Arch Otolaryngol Head Neck Surg* (2004) 130: 1411-1415.

[47] Morrison; PF; Laske, DW; Bobo, H; Oldfield, EH; Dedrick, RL. High-flow microinfusion: tissue penetration and pharmacodynamics. *Am J Physiol* (1994) 266: R292-305.

[48] Nierenberg, D; Harbaugh, R; Maurer, LH; Reeder, T; Scott, G; Fratkin, J; Newman, E. Continuous intratumoral infusion of methotrexate for recurrent glioblastoma: a pilot study. *Neurosurgery* (1991) 28: 752-761.

[49] Occhiogrosso, G; Edgar MA; Sandberg, DI; Souweidane, MM. Prolonged convection-enhanced delivery into the rat brainstem. *Neurosurgery* (2003) 52: 388-394.

[50] Olivi, A; Ewend, MG; Utsuki, T; Tyler, B, Domb, AJ; Brat, DJ; Brem, H. Interstitial delivery of carboplatin via biodegradable polymers is effective against experimental glioma in the rat. *Cancer Chemother Pharmacol* (1996) 39: 90-96.

[51] Packer, RJ; Krailo, M; Mehta, M; Warren, K; Allen, J, Jakachi, R; Villablanca, JG; Chiba, A; Reaman, G. Phase 1 study of concurrent RMP-7 and carboplatin with radiotherapy for children with newly diagnosed brainstem gliomas. *Cancer* (2005) Aug 2 [Epub ahead of print].

[52] Packer, RJ; Ater, J; Allen, J; Phillips, P; Geyer, R; Nicholson, HS; Jakacki, R; Kurczynski, E; Needle, M; Finlay, J; Reaman, G; Boyett, JM. Carboplatin and vincristine chemotherapy for children with newly diagnosed progressive low-grade gliomas. *J Neurosurg* (1997) 86: 747-754.

[53] Parney, IF; Kunwar, S; McDermott, M; Berger, M; Prados, M; Cha, S; Croteau, D; Puri, RK; Chang, SM. Neuroradiographic changes following convection-enhanced delivery of the recombinant cytotoxin interleukin 13-PE38QQR for recurrent malignant glioma. *J Neurosurg* (2005) 102: 267-275.

[54] Paxinos, G; Watson, C. *The rat brain in stereotaxic coordinates.* 2nd edn.. Academic Press Australia, North Ryde, N.S.W., Australia; 1986.

[55] Peterson, K; Harsh, G 4th; Fisher, PG; Adler, J; Le, Q. Daily low-dose carboplatin as a radiation sensitizer for newly diagnosed malignant glioma. *J Neuro-Oncol* (2001) 53: 27-32.

[56] Pollina, J; Plunkett, RJ; Ciesielski, MJ; Lis, A; Barone, TA; Greenberg, SJ; Fenstermaker, RA. Intratumoral infusion of topotecan prolongs survival in the nude rat intracranial U87 human glioma model. *J Neuro-Oncol* (1998) 39: 217-225.

[57] Prados, M; Lang, FF; Sherman, JW; Strauss, LC; Fleming, CK; Aldape, K; Kunwar, S; Yung, WKA; Chang, SM; Husain, SR; Gutin, PH; Raizer, J; Piepmeier, JM; Berger, M; McDermott, M; Puri, RK. Convection-enhanced delivery (CED) by positive pressure infusion of IL13-PE38QQR a recombinant tumor-targeted cytotoxin in recurrent malignant glioma. *Neuro-Oncol* (2002) 4 (suppl 1): S78.

[58] Prados, MD; Schold, SC JR SC; Fine, HA; Jaeckle, K; Hochberg, F; Mechtler, L; Fetell, MR.; Phuphanich, S; Feun, L; Janus, TJ; Ford, K; Graney, W. A randomized, double-blind, placebo-controlled, phase 2 study of RMP-7 in combination with carboplatin administered intraveneously for the treatment of recurrent malignant glioma. *Neuro-Oncol* (2003) 5: 96-103.

[59] Rosenberg, GA; Kyner, WT; Estrada, E. Bulk flow of brain interstitial fluid under normal and hyperosmolar conditions. *Am J Physiol* (1980) 238: F42-F49.

[60] Sandberg, DI; Edgar, MA; Souweidane, MM. Convection-enhanced delivery into the rat brainstem. *J Neurosurg* (2002) 96: 885-891.

[61] Sandberg, DI; Edgar, MA; Souweidane, MM. Effect of hyperosmolar mannitol on convection-enhanced delivery into the rat brain stem. *J Neuro-Oncol* (2002) 58: 187-192.

[62] Schabet, M; Martos, J; Buchholz, R; Pietsch, T. Animal models of human medulloblastoma: clinical, magnetic resonance imaging, and histopathological findings after intra-cisternal injection of MHH-MED-1 cells into nude rats. *Med Pediatr Oncol* (1997) 29: 92-97.

[63] Souweidane, MM; Occhiogrosso, G; Mark, EB; Edgar, MA; Dunkel, IJ. Interstitial infusion of carmustine in the rat brain stem with systemic administration of O^6-benzylguanine. *J Neuro-Oncol* (2004) 67: 319-326.

[64] Souweidane, MM; Occhiogrosso, G; Mark, EB; Edgar, MA. Interstitial infusion of IL13-PE38QQR in the rat brainstem. *J Neuro-Oncol* (2004) 67: 1021-1029.

[65] Storm, PB; Clatterbuck, RE; Liu, JY; Johnson, RM; Gillis, EM; Guarnieri, M; Carson, BS. A surgical technique for safely placing a drug delivery catheter into the pons of primates: preliminary results of carboplatin infusion. *Neurosurgery* (2003) 52: 1169-1177.

[66] Strege, RJ; Liu, YJ; Kiely, A; Johnson, RM; Gillis, EM; Storm, P; Carson, BS; Jallo, GI; Guarnieri, M. Toxicity and cerebrospinal fluid levels of carboplatin chronically infused into the brainstem of a primate. *J Neuro-Oncol* (2004) 67: 327-334.

[67] Valtonen, S; Timonen, U; Toivanen, P; Kalimo, H; Kivipelto, L; Heiskanen, O; Unsgaard, G; Kuurne, T. Interstitial chemotherapy with carmustine-loaded polymers for high-grade gliomas: a randomized double-blind study. *Neurosurgery* (1997) 41: 44-49.

[68] Viola, JJ; Agbaria, R; Walbridge, S; Oshiro, EM; Johns, DG; Kelley, JA; Oldfield, EH; Ram, Z. In situ cyclopentenyl cytosine infusion for the treatment of experimental brain tumors. *Cancer Res* (1995) 55: 1306-1309.

[69] Vogelbaum, MA. Convection enhanced delivery for the treatment of malignant gliomas: symposium review. *J Neuro-Oncol* (2005) 73: 57-69.

[70] Walker, DA; Punt, JAG; Sokal, M. Clinical management of brain stem glioma. *Arch Dis Child* (1999) 80: 558-564.

[71] Warren, KE; Patel, MC; Atkin, AA; Widemann, B; Libucha, M; Adamson, PC; Neuwirth, R; Benziger, D; O'Toole, T; Ford, K; Patronas, N; Packer, RJ; Balis, FM. Phase I trial of lobradimil (RMP-7) and carboplatin in children with brain tumors. *Cancer Chemother Pharmacol* (2001) 48: 275-282.

[72] Weingart, JD; Strauss, L; Grossman, S; Markert, J; Tatter, S; Fisher, J; Fleming, C; Puri, R. Phase I/II study: intratumoral infusion of IL13-PE38QQR cytotoxin for recurrent supratentorial malignant glioma. *Neuro-Oncology* (2002) 4: 379.

[73] Westphal, M; Black, PMcL. Perspectives of cellular and molecular neurosurgery. *J Neuro-Oncol* (2004) 70: 255-269.

[74] Wu, Q; Tyler, B; Sukay, L; Rhines, L; DiMeco, F; Clatterbuck, RE; Guarnieri, M, Carson, BS. Experimental rodent models of brainstem tumors. *Vet Pathol* (2002) 39: 293-299.

[75] Wu, Q; Guarnieri, M; Tyler, B; Clatterbuck, RE; Liu, Y; Carson, BS. Section on tumors: young investigator award: local release of carboplatin via an Alzet mini-osmotic pump prolongs survival in a rat brainstem tumor model. *Clin Neurosurg* (2004) 51: 332-339.

[76] Yachnis, AT. Neuropathology of pediatric brain tumors. *Semin Pediatr Neurol* (1997) 4: 282-291.

[77] Zanotti, KM; Rybicki, LA; Kennedy, AW; Belinson, JL; Webster, KD; Kulp, B; Peterson, G; Markman, M. Carboplatin skin testing: a skin-testing protocol for

predicting hypersensitivity to carboplatin chemotherapy. *J Clin Oncol* (2001) 19: 3126-3129.

In: Brain Cancer: Therapy and Surgical Interventions... ISBN 1-59454-974-5
Editor: Andrew V. Yang, pp. 45-75

Chapter III

Antitumoural Action of Neurokinin-1 Receptor Antagonists on Human Brain Cancer Cell Lines

M. Muñoz[1*], M. Rosso[1], R. Coveñas[2] and J. A. Soult[1]
[1] Pediatric Intensive Care Unit,
"Virgen del Rocío" University Children's Hospital, Sevilla, Spain
[2] Laboratory of Neuroanatomy of the Peptidergic Systems,
Institute of Neurosciences of Castilla y León, Salamanca, Spain

Abstract

Substance P is an undecapeptide that belongs to the tachykinin family of peptides and has a widespread distribution in both the central and peripheral nervous systems. It is known that substance P, neurokinin A, neuropeptide K and neuropeptide Gamma are derived from the preprotachykinin A gene, whereas neurokinin B is derived from the preprotachykinin B gene. The biological actions of substance P, neurokinin A and neurokinin B are mediated by three receptors, designated neurokinin (NK)-1, NK-2 and NK-3, the biological action of substance P being preferentially mediated by the NK1 receptor. After binding to the NK1 receptor, substance P regulates many biological functions, and this neuropeptide has also been implicated in inflammation, pain and depression.

Preclinical investigations have shown that activation of the NK1 receptor by substance P induces mitogenesis in several human tumour cell lines, and that NK1 receptor antagonists (e.g., L-733,060) display antitumoural action against human cancer cell lines (glioma, retinoblastoma, neuroblastoma...). In addition, it has been documented that astrocytomas and gliomas contain significant levels of NK1 receptors and that both

* Full Address: Dr. Miguel Muñoz; Hospital Infantil Virgen del Rocío, Unidad de Cuidados Intensivos Pediátricos, Av. Manuel Siurot s/n, 41013 – Sevilla, Spain; Phone number: 34-955012965; E-mail: mmunoz@cica.es; Fax number: 34-955012921

express substance P. Thus, the development of antagonist molecules of the NK1 receptor represents an important opportunity for exploiting these molecules as novel therapeutic agents. The antitumoural action of one of these antagonists (L-733,060) (estimated affinity = 0.8 nM) has been tested in several cancer cell lines (glioma, neuroblastoma, retinoblastoma...), but the antitumoural action of other NK1 receptor antagonists (e.g., L-732,138) is unknown.

Accordingly, the aim of this study, using the tetrazolium compound [3-(4,5-dimethylthiazol-2-yl)-5-(3-carboxymethoxyphenyl)2-(4-sulfophenyl)-2H-tetrazolium], inner salt, a colorimetric method to evaluate cell viability, was to demonstrate the antitumoural action of the potent and highly selective competitive NK1 receptor antagonist L-732,138 (N-acetyl-L-tryptophan 3, 5-bis(trifluoromethyl) benzyl ester) (IC_{50} = 2.3 nM) on the GAMG glioma cell line and compare its antitumoural action with those previously reported in the same tumour cell line after using the selective, potent and long-acting non-peptide tachykinin NK1 receptor antagonist L-733,060. In addition, here we review the data currently available about the action of substance P and NK1 receptor antagonists in human cancer cell lines (glioma, astrocytoma, retinoblastoma...). The following aspects are discussed: 1) Substance P and the NK1 receptor; 2) Mitogenic action of substance P; 3) NK1 receptor antagonists; 4) Antitumoural action of L-732,138 on the human GAMG glioma cell line; 5) Antitumoural action of NK1 receptor antagonists; 6) Substance P, inflammation, pain and cancer; 7) Substance P, psychiatric disorders and cancer: possible relationship between the progression of cancer and cerebral mechanisms; 8) Possible clinical implications of NK1 receptor antagonists; 9) Future research on NK1 receptor antagonists.

The data suggest that NK1 receptor antagonists act as a broad-spectrum antitumoural agent and that they could be a promising therapeutic drug for the treatment of human brain tumours.

Key words: Glioma; Astrocytoma; Retinoblastoma; Substance P; NK1 receptor; L-732,138; L-733,060

Introduction

In recent years, the expression and secretion of peptides by tumours has gained increasing interest since these peptides have been shown to influence tumour proliferation. Thus, it has been demonstrated that substance P acts through the neurokinin-1 (NK1) receptor as a mitogen on several human cancer cell lines (glioma, retinoblastoma, neuroblastoma) (see Muñoz et al., 2005a, b). In addition, receptors for several peptides (somatostatin, galanin, substance P, cholecystokinin...) have been observed in a wide variety of tumours (see Reubi, 2003; Berger et al., 2005; Muñoz et al., 2005a) and NK1 receptor antagonists (e.g., L-733,060...) show antitumoural activity against human cancer cell lines, including tumoural brain cell lines (see Muñoz et al., 2004a, 2005a). All the above data suggest that the substance P/NK1 receptor system could play an important role in the development of cancer; that substance P may be a universal mitogen in NK1 receptor-expressing tumour cell types; that NK1 receptor antagonists act as a broad-spectrum antitumoural agent, and that they could be a promising therapeutic drug for the treatment of human cancer (including brain tumours).

Finally, the results suggest that the NK1 receptor may be a new and promising target in the treatment of human cancer cell lines.

Other strategies different from treatment with NK1 receptor antagonists (see Muñoz et al., 2004a, b, 2005 a, b) have been applied against tumour cells. Thus for example, the treatment of tumours by using peptide analogues labelled with cytotoxic agents acting via specific receptors has been tested for neuropeptide Y (Koglin and Beck-Sickinger, 2004). However, this action is dependent on the ability of the peptide to internalise upon receptor-ligand interaction on the cell surface.

The majority of intracraneal tumours arise from brain parenchyma, primarily from glial cells (astrocytes or oligodendrocytes). Primary neuronal tumours are uncommon. Meningeal tumours are the second most common type of intracranial tumour. Tumours also arise from a variety of other cell types, including some not normally found in the brain, such as germ cells, lymphocytes and remains of embryonic tissues (Kleihues and Cavanee, 2000). Brain metastases are much more common than primary intracraneal tumours; aproximately 170,000 people in the USA are diagnosed with brain mestastases every year. In children and men aged 20-39 years, brain tumours are the second leading cause of cancer-related death (Wrensch et al., 2002).

According to the World Health Organization (Kleihues and Cavanee, 2000), tumours in the nervous system can be histologically classified in:

A. *Neuroepithelial tumours*
   1. Astrocytic tumours
      - Pilocytic astrocytoma (WHO grade I)
      - Diffuse astrocytoma (WHO grade II)
      - Anaplastic astrocytoma (WHO grade III)
      - Glioblastoma multiforme (WHO grade IV)
      - Pleomorphic xanthoastrocytoma
      - Subependymal giant cell astrocytoma
   2. Oligondendroglial tumours:
      - Oligondendroglioma, low-grade or anaplastic
   3. Ependymal tumours
      - Ependymoma, low-grade or anaplastic
      - Subependymoma
      - Myxopapillary ependymoma
   4. Choroid plexus tumours
      - Choroid plexus papilloma
      - Choroid plexus carcinoma
   5. Neuronal/mixed glial-neuronal tumours
   6. Pineal parenchymal tumours
   7. Embryonal tumours
      - Meduloepithelioma
      - Ependymoblastoma
      - Meduloblastoma
      - Primitive neuroectodermal tumour (PNET):

- Neuroblastoma
- Ganglioneuroblastoma

8. Neuroblastic tumours
   - Olfactory neuroblastoma
   - Olfactory neuroepithelioma
   - Neuroblastoma of the adrenal gland and of the sympathetic nervous system

B. Meningeal tumours

1. Meningioma
2. Hemangiopericytoma
3. Melanocytoma

C. Tumours of cranial nerves

D. Germ cell tumours

F. Primary central nervous system lymphoma

G. Tumours of the sellar region

H. Cysts and tumour-like lesions

I. Metastastic tumours

The retina is an "approachable part of the brain "whose circuitry is particularly amenable to study. Unlike the other sensory organs found in the periphery, the retina itself is part of the central nervous system; embryologically, it is formed from the optic cup, an outpouching of the neural tube. The retina has much in common with the rest of the central nervous system (such as neurotransmitter and receptor families), but is far easier to study in vitro (Reid, 1999). Retinoblastoma is a malignant tumour of the retina, usually arising in the inner nuclear layer of the neural retina. Retinoblastoma is unusual in being caused by an autosomal dominant mutation in some cases (about 6%), in which case it may be bilateral. The gene product of the retinoblastoma gene is a tumour suppressor that interacts with transcription factors such as E2F to block transcription of growth-regulating genes (Lackie and Dow, 1995).

In this paper, we shall focus our review and study on the actions of substance P and NK1 receptor antagonists in some human central nervous system cancer cell lines (glioma, astrocytoma, retinoblastoma).

Gliomas are the most serious brain tumours in adult. They arise from glial cells and infiltrate the brain diffusely. They are derived from three basic types of glial cells: astrocytes, ependimocytes and oligodendrocytes, and together account for 67.6% of all primary brain tumours. Astrocytes are the most numerous of the glial cells and subserve a number of functions including metabolic support to neurons and the induction/formation of the blood-brain barrier. Astrocyte gliomas are the most common type and include anaplastic astrocytomas, accounting for 10-30% of all gliomas, in individuals aged 35-55 years, with median survival of 24-36 months, and the highly malignant glioblastoma multiforme, which can arise de novo or from pre-existing low-grade astrocytoma, with a accounts for 45-50% of all gliomas, frequently in individuals aged 45-65 years, with a median survival of approximately 9-12 months. The prognosis for patients with malignant gliomas is mostly influenced by histological grade and age (see Fine, 1994).

Retinoblastoma arises from the photoreceptor elements, poorly differentiated neuroblasts, of the inner layer of the retina (Perentes et al., 1987). This tumour comprises 3% of tumours recorded in children younger than the age of 15 years and represents one of the most common malignant tumours of childhood, with an incidence of 1 in 15,000 live births and an increased frequency in patients with a positive family history of retinoblastoma (Tamboli et al., 1990; Shields and Shields, 1999). The malignancy leads to metastatic disease and death in 50% of children worldwide, but in less 5% of children in developed nations with advanced medical care (Shields and Shields, 2004). Several methods are currently being developed to improve the success rates of eye preservation (60%) with useful visual functions (Kaneko and Suzuki, 2003).

The past decade has witnessed an exponential increase in research into cancer. This has led to a considerable increase in investment in the field. This effort, however, has not been translated in better perspectives as regards the problem, although several fields of research have been promising, such as the human genome project, gene therapy, the search for new cytostatic agents and stem cell research. The short- and medium-term perspectives are not very promising and hence now pathways must be opened up to offer future hope to oncologic patients. In this sense, it is expected that in the near future newer and more effective and safe anticancer drugs will become available for the treatment of central nervous system tumours. One of these treatments could involve NK1 receptor antagonists.

Thus, the present review summarizes current knowledge of the mitogenic action of substance P and the antitumoural action of NK1 receptor antagonists on some human central nervous system cancer cells, such as glioma, astrocytoma and retinoblastoma. Another aim of this study, using the tetrazolium compound [3-(4,5-dimethylthiazol-2-yl)-5-(3-carboxymethoxyphenyl)2-(4-sulfophenyl)-2H-tetrazolium], inner salt, a colorimetric method to evaluate cell viability, was to demonstrate the antitumoural action of the potent and highly selective competitive NK1 receptor antagonist L-732,138 (N-acetyl-L-tryptophan 3,5-bis(trifluoromethyl)benzyl ester) (IC_{50} = 2.3 nM) on the GAMG glioma cell line and compare its antitumoural action with those previously reported in the same tumour cell line, using the selective, potent and long-acting non-peptide tachykinin NK1 receptor antagonist L-733,060 (Muñoz et al., 2004a, 2005a).

Substance P and the NK1 Receptor

Substance P (SP) is an undecapeptide that belongs to the tachykinin family of peptides (this family also includes peptides such as neurokinin A, neurokinin B, kassinin, ranakinin, eledoisin, neuropeptide K and neuropeptide Gamma). It is also known that SP, neurokinin A, neuropeptide K and neuropeptide Gamma are derived from the preprotachykinin A gene, whereas neurokinin B is derived from the preprotachykinin B gene.

A large number of immunohistochemical and radioimmunological studies have been carried out on the distribution of SP in the mammalian central and peripheral nervous systems (Cuello and Kanazawa, 1978; Hökfelt et al., 1978; Mai et al., 1986; Burgos et al., 1988). All these studies have shown that this neuropeptide has a widespread distribution in both the central and the peripheral nervous systems.

SP is a neuroactive substance that elicits excitatory effects as a neurotransmitter or neuromodulator in the nervous system; that it is hydrolysed, for example, by endopeptidase-24.11 (Turner, 1987), and that it has been well characterized not only in terms of distribution but also as regards the sites of its release and its biological actions. After binding to the NK1 receptor, SP regulates many biological functions (von Euler and Gaddum, 1931; Pernow, 1983; Hökfelt et al., 2001). Thus, SP has been implicated, for example, in the regulation of the cardiovascular system, in the dilatation of the arterial system, in neuronal survival and degeneration, in the regulation of respiratory mechanisms, in sensory perception, in movement control, in gastric movility, in salivation and in micturition (Unger et al., 1981; see Hershey et al., 1991; see Quartara and Maggi, 1998). This neuropeptide has also been implicated in inflammation, pain and depression (Rupniak et al., 1996; Kramer et al., 1998; Samsam et al., 2000; Harrison and Geppetti, 2001; Bang et al., 2003; Varty et al., 2003). Moreover, SP has also been found in human neuroblastoma cells of the parotid gland (Shrestha et al., 1994); it is expressed in almost 90% of metastatic neuroblastoma cells in the bone marrow (Nowicki and Miskowiak, 2002), and it has been documented in human malignant gliomas (Palma et al., 1999, 2000) and retinoblastoma (Tarkkanen et al., 1983).

The biological actions of SP, neurokinin A and neurokinin B are mediated by three receptors, designated neurokinin NK1, NK2 and NK3, the biological action of SP being preferentially mediated by the NK1 receptor, since SP is the natural ligand with the highest affinity for the NK1 receptor. Thus, the NK1 receptor is defined as a the mediator of the biological activities encoded by the C-terminal sequence of tachykinins, for which SP is a more potent agonist than neurokinin A or neurokinin B (see Quartara and Maggi, 1997). The NK1 receptor is functionally coupled with G-protein (MacDonald and Boyd, 1989).

The distribution of the NK1 receptor in the mammalian central nervous system has been carried out by autoradiography, by studying the expression of the mRNA encoding for the NK1 receptor protein and by immunocytochemistry (Wolf et al., 1985; Dam and Quirion, 1986; Danks et al., 1986; Saffroy et al, 1988; Maeno et al., 1993; Nakaya et al., 1994; Whitty et al., 1995). These studies revealed a widespread distribution of the NK1 receptor in the mammalian central nervous system and in peripheral tissues. Furthermore, it has been demonstrated that the NK1 receptor expression is increased 25-36-fold in human pancreatic cancer cell lines in comparison with normal controls, and that tumours samples of patients with advanced tumour stages exhibit significantly higher NK1 receptor levels (see Friess et al., 2003). In addition, the number of NK1 receptors expressed in the human normal cells is lower (e.g., human blood T-lymphocytes express 7,000-10,000 NK1 receptors/cell) (Payan et al. 1986) than that expressed in human tumoural cells (e.g., astrocytoma cells express 40,000 NK1 receptors/cell) (Fowler et al., 1994). It is also known that high levels of NK1 receptors are expressed in human glioma cell lines U373 MG (Palma et al., 1999) and UC11 MG (Johnson et al., 1991), as well as that human glioma GAMG and neuroblastoma SKN-BE(2) cell lines expressed NK1 receptors (Muñoz et al., 2005a). Moreover, an increased percentage of NK1 receptor expression in astrocytoma and glioblastoma tumours possessing the most malignant phenotypes has been reported (Hennig et al., 1995) and that SP induces cell proliferation in several cancer cell lines after the activation of NK1 receptors (Muñoz et al., 2004b, 2005a, b).

The stimulation of NK1 receptors can generate several second messengers which, in turn, can trigger a wide range of effector mechanisms that are responsible for regulating cellular excitability and function. Three second-messenger systems have been reported to be activated following NK1 receptor occupancy by agonists: a) stimulation, via phospholipase C, of phosphatidyl inositol turnover, leading to Ca mobilization from both intra- and extracellular sources; b) arachidonic acid mobilization via phospholipase A2; and c) cAMP accumulation via stimulation of adenylate cyclase (Mitsuhashi et al., 1992; Nakajima et al., 1992; Takeda et al., 1992; Seabrook and Fong, 1993; García et al., 1994; Mochizuki-Oda et al., 1994). In addition, it has been demonstrated that the activation of NK1 receptors by SP or by its agonists produces in human astrocytoma U373 MG and UC11 MG cell lines the following actions: induces the activation of phospholipase D, the formation of inositol phosphates and the release of interleukins (IL-8 and IL-6), taurine and glutamate, it mobilizes intracellular calcium, it influences both glutamate and K^+ transport, and it stimulates glycogen breakdown (Johnson et al., 1991; Lee et al., 1992; Johnson and Johnson, 1993; Bordey et al., 1994; Medrano et al., 1994; Oury-Donat et al., 1994; Palma and Manzini, 1998; Torrens et al., 1998).

The pharmacological profile of NK1 receptors is similar in human lymphoblastoma and astrocytoma cells; i.e., if NK1 receptor subtypes exist in humans, these cell lines are likely to express a similar subtype (Goso et al., 1994). Moreover, several previous reports have shown that different isoforms of the NK1 receptor can be found in both human and rat tissues (Caberlotto et al., 2003). For instance, in human lymphocytes a glycosylated NK1 receptor of 58 kDa is found (McGillis et al, 1990), whereas this form and two others of 38 kDa and 33 kDa respectively are also present in IM-9 lymphoblasts (Organist et al., 1988; van Ginkel et al., 1996). In rat tissues, several NK1 receptor forms have been detected, with sizes ranging from 54 kDa to 46 kDa (Nakata et al., 1988; van Ginkel et al., 1996), whereas the presence of NK1 receptors in both neuroblastoma SKN-BE(2) and glioma GAMG cell lines has also been demonstrated (Muñoz et al., 2005a). Thus, in this latter study different isoforms of the NK1 receptor were reported in both neuroblastoma SKN-BE(2) and glioma GAMG cell lines. Whereas in the SKN-BE(2) cell line a major 54 kDa band is observed, in GAMG cells two additional and more abundant isoforms of about 38 and 33 kDa are detected. However, at present, the functional roles of the different isoforms of the NK1 receptor in both human cancer cells are unknown.

Finally, it has been reported that upon exposure to the agonist SP, this peptide and its receptor are internalized into early endosomes within minutes of binding, these events being observed both in vivo and in vitro (Bowden et al, 1994; Garland et al., 1994; Grady et al, 1995; Mantyh et al., 1995). The loss of NK1 receptors from the cell membrane is blocked by inhibition of clathrin-mediated endocytosis. Recovery of NK1 receptor expression at membrane level requires endosomal acidification but not novel protein synthesis. Internalized SP is intact in early endosomes but is slowly degraded in perinuclear vesicles (Grady et al., 1995). Thus, SP induces a clathrin-dependent internalization of the NK1 receptor; the SP/NK1 receptor complex dissociates in acidified endosomes, and SP is then degraded, whereas the NK1 receptor recycles at the cell surface (Grady et al, 1995).

Mitogenic Action of Substance P

It is known that SP stimulates mitogenesis by activating NK1 receptors in several normal (Payan et al., 1983; Nilsson et al., 1985; Lotz et al., 1987; Ziche et al., 1990) and tumoural cell types, probably via autocrine/paracrine mechanisms (Luo et al., 1996; Sharif et al., 1996; Palma et al., 1999; Muñoz et al., 2004b, 2005a, b). It is also known that SP is expressed in almost 90% of metastatic human neuroblastoma cells (Nowicki and Miskowiak, 2002) and retinoblastoma (Tarkkanen et al., 1983), and that the NK1 receptor is expressed in U373 MG, U138 MG, UC11 MG and GAMG human glioma cell lines, as well as in astrocytoma (Fowler and Brannstrom, 1994; Palma et al., 1999, 2000; Muñoz et al., 2005a) and neuroblastoma (Muñoz et al., 2005a). In addition, it has been reported that more astrocytoma/glioma primary tumours express the NK1 receptor than do established astrocytoma/glioma cell lines in culture (Luo et al., 1996).

In addition, a mitogenic role for SP in amphibian limb regeneration has been described (Globus et al., 1991), and it has been reported that SP is a mitogen in mammalian connective tissue cells (Nilsson et al., 1985), in regenerating planarians (Salo and Baguna, 1986) and in human melanoma cell lines (Muñoz et al., 2004b). Moreover, it has been reported that substance K, an elongated form of neurokinin A, induces mitogenesis (Nilsson et al., 1985; Cyr et al., 1991; Sharif et al., 1996). Finally, the galanin receptor has been shown to exhibit mitogenic signalling properties via the MAP kinase pathway, which plays an important role in cell proliferation (Hammond et al., 1996; Seufferlein and Rozengurt, 1996).

In several glial brain tumour-derived cell lines, the presence of NK1 receptors is strictly correlated with the effect of SP and/or neurokinin A on increases in DNA synthesis and cellular proliferation (Luo et al., 1996; Sharif et al., 1996; Palma at al., 1999). Thus, for example, previous studies analysing the role of SP in inducing mitogenesis in the human astrocytoma cell line U-373 MG have been published (Lee et al., 1989; Eistetter et al., 1992; Luo et al., 1996). One of them reports that activation of the NK1 receptor has no significant effect on DNA synthesis (Lee et al., 1989). In contrast, the other studies show that activation of the NK1 receptor by nanomolar concentrations of SP induces DNA synthesis and mitogenesis in the astrocytoma cell line U-373 MG (Eistetter et al., 1992; Luo et al., 1996). This observation is in agreement with the findings reported by other authors, since it has been observed that SP stimulates the mitogenesis of GAMG cells (this cell line has NK1 receptors) (Muñoz et al., 2005a), since after administration of SP a proliferation of the GAMG glioma cell line is observed. It is known that SP acts specifically through the NK1 receptor in this cancer cell line, because L-733,060 (an NK1 receptor antagonist) growth inhibition of GAMG cells is partially reversed by administration of a nanomolar dose of exogenous SP (Muñoz et al., 2005a). This is also the case of the human neuroblastoma SKN-BE(2) cell line and the human retinoblastoma WERI-Rb-1 and Y-79 cell lines, since growth inhibition of these three cancer cell lines is also partially reversed by administration of a nanomolar dose of exogenous SP (Muñoz et al., 2005a, b).

Finally, it should be added that in addition to SP several other substances have been identified as crucial in the biology of gliomas, exerting their effects on cellular proliferation and differentiation through intracellular signalling mechanisms (Maxwell et al., 1990; Schlegel et al., 1990; Takahashi et al., 1990; Plate et al., 1992; Stockhammer et al., 1995).

In sum, the above data suggest that activation of NK1 receptors induces mitogenesis in human astrocytoma (Luo et al., 1996), glioma (Palma et al., 1999, 2000; Muñoz et al., 2005a), neuroblastoma (Muñoz et al., 2005a), retinoblastoma (Muñoz et al., 2005b) and melanoma cells (Muñoz et al., 2004b), an effect involving the expression of the c-myc protein and tyrosine kinase signalling (Luo et al., 1996).

NK1 Receptor Antagonists

Important advances have been made in the development of highly selective agonists and antagonists for the NK1 receptor in order to better know the physiological actions of SP and the pathophysiological significance of NK1 receptors.

It has been suggested that NK1 receptor antagonists, at the level of the central nervous system, could be used to produce analgesia, antidepressive, anxiolytic and antiemetic effects, and for the treatment of certain forms of urinary incontinence due to detrusor hyperreflexia. In the peripheral nervous system, NK1 receptor antagonists could be used in several inflammatory diseases including arthritis, inflammatory bowel diseases and cystitis (see Quartara and Maggi, 1998). Below we report a list of some of the peptide and non-peptide NK1 receptor antagonists to be found in the literature.

I. Peptide Antagonist

During the last decade, research and development of small molecules as antagonists of the NK1 receptor have represented an important opportunity for the development of novel therapeutic agents. Most of the work done in the design and preparation of antagonists for the NK1 receptor has focused on the introduction of D-amino acids (Almeida et al., 2004). Thus, several peptide antagonists derived from SP have been developed, since the first non-peptide NK1 receptor antagonist CP-96,345 was developed (Snider et al., 1990). However, their affinity is several orders of magnitude lower than that of natural agonists, as well as the metabolic instability and the inability to gain access to the central nervous system through the blood-brain barrier of peptide NK1 receptor antagonists limits their usefulness for in vivo studies. In addition, in general these substances suffer from a number of drawbacks, such as poor potency and ability to discriminate between tachykinin receptors, partial residual agonist activity, mast cell degranulating activity and neurotoxicity after administration in the central nervous system (Lee et al., 1986; see Quartara and Maggi, 1997).

Some of these peptide NK1 antagonists are listed below:

- [D-Arg^1, D-$Trp^{7,9}$, Leu^{11}] SP (Spantide I). This antagonist is neurotoxic and a potent histamine releaser from mast cells.
- H-D-Lys(Nicotinoyl)-Pro-[3-(3-pyridyl)-Ala]-pro-D-Phe83,4-Cl_2)-Asn-D- Trp-Phe-D-Trp-Leu-Nle-NH_2 (Spantide II). This antagonist is devoid of neurotoxicity (Folkers et al., 1990).
- [D-Arg^1, D-$Trp^{5,7,9}$, Leu^{11}] SP

- [D-Arg^{1}, D-Pro^{2}, D-Trp ^{7,9}, Leu^{11}] SP
- [D-Arg^{1}, D-Phe^{5}, D-Trp^{7,9}, Leu^{11}] SP
- [Arg^{6}, D-Trp^{7,9}, MePhe^{8}] SP (6-11)
- [D-Pro^{2}- Trp^{7,9}] SP
- [D-Pro^{4}, D-Trp ^{7,9,10}, Phe^{11}] SP (4-11)
- p-HOPA-DTrp-Phe-DTrp-Leu-Leu-NH_2: NY-3238
- DMePhe-DTrp-Phe-DTrp-Leu(CH_2NH)Leu- NH_2: NY-3460

II. Non-peptide Antagonists

Since non-peptide NK1 receptor antagonists have become available (Maggi et al., 1993; Regoli et al., 1994), an increasing number of papers describing new non-peptide antagonists has been published (see Quartara and Maggi, 1997). Thus, steroids (WIN- 51,708...), perhydroisoindolones (RP-67,580, RP-73,467, RPR-100,893...), benzylamino and benzylether quinuclidine (CP-96,345, L-709,210...), benzylamino piperidines (CP-99,994, GR-203,040, GR-205,171, CP-122,721...), benzylether piperidines (L-733,060, L-741,671, L-742,694...) and tryptophan-based (L-732,138...) NK1 receptor antagonists have been reported (see Quartara and Maggi, 1997). The investigation into non-peptide NK1 receptor antagonists is a field that is developing very quickly. In the following, list other non-peptide tachykinin NK1 receptor antagonists, not mentioned above, are included:

- SR-1,400,333
- MEN-11,467
- MEN-11,149
- Vofopitant (GR-205,171)
- Ezlopitant (CJ-11,974)
- CJ-12,458 (active metabolite of Ezlopitant)
- CJ-12,764 (active metabolite of Ezlopitant)
- MK-869 (L-754,030)
- L-758,298
- L-759,274

L-733,060 is a selective, potent and long-acting central non-peptide tachykinin NK1 receptor antagonist showing high affinity for the human NK1 receptor in vitro (Rupniak et al., 1996). It belongs to the benzylether piperidine family of NK1 receptor antagonists (Harrison et al., 1994). It is known that the administration of L-733,060 produces analgesia (Rupniak et al., 1996) and antidepressive effects (Kramer et al., 1998; Varty et al., 2003), and the compound has been used in the treatment of a broad range of anxiety and mood disorders (Rupniak et al., 2000) and inflammatory liver disease, most likely by inhibiting the effects of SP (Bang et al., 2003). In addition, it has been reported that L-733,060 acts as an antitumoural agent on melanoma, glioma, neuroblastoma and retinoblastoma cell lines (Muñoz et al., 2004a, b; 2005a, b). In this sense, it would be very interesting to know whether the treatment of cancer cell lines with the NK1 receptor antagonists that have been studied so far in humans (Diemunsch and Grelot, 2000) may or may not produce the same growth inhibitory action as found with L-733,060. At present, there are more than thirty compounds that act as NK1 receptor antagonists (Giardina et al., 2003). In this study, we tested one of these NK1 receptor antagonists; namely L-732,138.

L-732,138 (N-acetyl-L-tryptophan 3,5-bis(trifluoromethyl) benzyl ester) shows a competitive and selective antagonism for the NK1 receptor. It is approximately 1000-fold more potent in cloned human NK1 receptors than in cloned human NK-2 and NK-3 receptors; and approximately 200-fold more potent in human NK1 receptors than in rat NK1 receptors (MacLeod et al., 1994). The IC_{50} for the human NK1 receptor expressed in CHO cells is approximately 2.3 nM (Cascieri et al., 1994). It is known that the administration of L-732,138 produces an attenuation of hyperalgesia (Cahill and Coderre, 2002) and it has been described that L-732,138 is able to antagonize H(3) antagonist-induced skin vascular permeability (Hossen et al., 2003). Currently, the possible antitumoural action of the tryptophan-based antagonist L-732,138 is unknown. In the next section, we shall discuss the antitumoural action of this NK1 receptor antagonist against the GAMG glioma cell line.

Antitumoural Action of L-732,138 on the Human GAMG Glioma Cell Line

Cell Cultures

We used the human glioma cell line GAMG (Deutsche Sammlung von Mikroorganismen und Zellkulturen [DSMZ] Braunschweig, Germany) (see Figures 1 and 2).

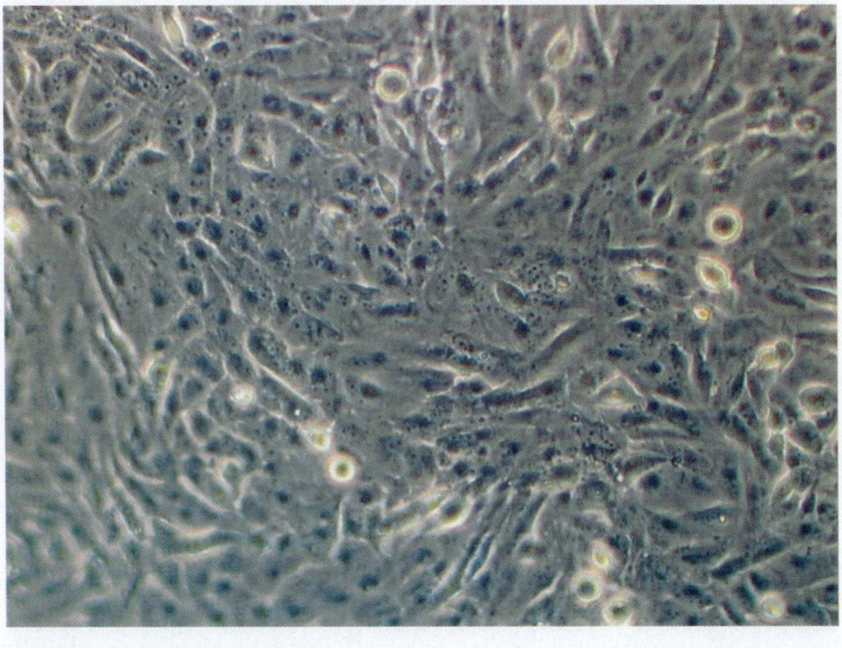

Figure 1. GAMG cells in culture (x 40).

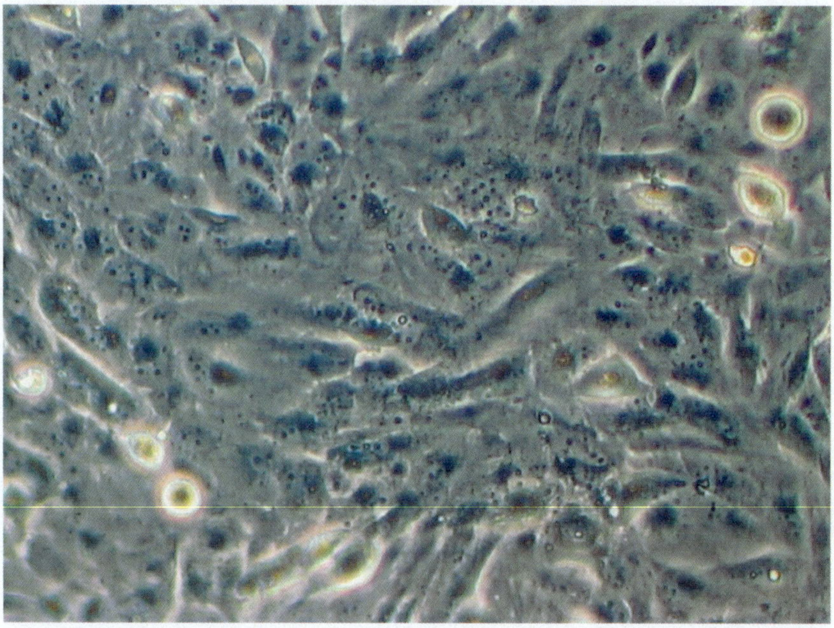

Figure 2. GAMG cells in culture. Here, a high-power image of Figure 1 can be observed (x 60).

The GAMG cell line was maintained in Dulbecco´s MEM supplemented with 10% heat-inactivated foetal bovine serum, according to the culture conditions suggested by the ATCC (American Type Culture Collection) and DSMZ. The cell line was seeded in 75 cm^2 tissue culture flasks (Falcon, Heidelberg, Germany). The medium was renewed every two days and the cells were harvested by treatment with trypsin (0.05% and 0.02% EDTA without Ca^{2+} and Mg^{2+}) on the sixth day after seeding. Cells were incubated at 37° C in a humidified atmosphere (95% air/5% CO_2).

Drug Treatments

SP (Arg-Pro-Lys-Pro-Gln-Gln-Phe-Phe-Gly-Leu-Met-NH_2) acetate salt (Sigma-Aldrich, Madrid, Spain) was dissolved in distilled water. The NK1 receptor antagonist N-acetyl-L-tryptophan 3, 5-bis (trifluoromethyl) benzyl ester (L-732,138) (Sigma-Aldrich, Madrid, Spain), MW 472.39, was dissolved in distilled water containing 0.2% dimethylsulphoxide (DMSO) before sample treatment. GAMG cells were treated with 10, 20, 40 and 100 μM of L-732,138 (Figure 3). Moreover, different concentrations of SP (10, 50 and 100 nM) were evaluated (Figure 4). Finally, the most mitogen-effective SP concentration for the GAMG cell line (50 nM) (see Figure 4) was incubated 1 h before the addition of L-732,138 (20 μM).

Proliferation Assays

Cell proliferation was evaluated using the tetrazolium compound 3-(4,5-dimethylthiazol-2-yl)-5-(3-carboxymethoxyphenyl)2-(4-sulfophenyl)-2H-tetrazolium, inner salt (MTS), according to the manufacturer's instructions (CellTiter 96 Aqueous One-Solution Cell Proliferation Assay, Promega Corp., Madison, USA). At the time of the assays, cells cultured for 4-5 days were harvested by trypsinization, and cell viability was evaluated by Trypan blue exclusion. Cell numbers were quantified using a Coulter counter. Cells were cultured in 96-well plates, each well containing 10^4 cells in a total volume of 100 μl. The plates included blank wells (0 cells/0.1 ml), control wells (10^4 cells/0.1 ml), control wells with DMSO, control wells treated with L-732,138 at different concentrations, and control wells treated with the most effective SP concentration and L-732,138. The plates were inoculated with L-732,138 (10, 20, 40 and 100 μM) and were incubated for a period (first doubling time) of 48 h (Figure 3). Other plates were inoculated with exogenous SP (10, 50 and 100 nM). As it is shown in Figure 4, SP-induced cell proliferation. In addition, the most effective SP concentration (50 nM) for the GAMG cell line was added to the plates, containing the glioma GAMG cell line, 1 h before the addition of L-732,138 (20 μM) (Figure 4).

For proliferation assays, 20 μl of MTS reagent was added to each well 90 min before reading the samples in a multiscanner microplate reader (TECAN Spectra classic, Barcelona, Spain) at 492 nm. The quantity of product, as measured by optical density, was directly proportional to the number of living cells. Each experimental condition was assayed in duplicate and all experiments were performed at least three times. The fifty-percent inhibition concentration (IC_{50}) of L-732,138 was calculated using a curve-fitting parameter.

Statistical Analyses

The data were evaluated statistically using Student's *t*-test, taking $p \leq 0.01$ as the level of significance.

Growth inhibition of the GAMG glioma cell line by L-732,138 was observed after the addition of increasing concentrations of L-732,138 (Figure 3). Treatment of the GAMG cell line with L-732,138 resulted in a concentration-dependent cytotoxicity (see Figure 3). Thus, the concentration required for a 50% reduction in optical density (IC_{50}) observed in the controls treated with L-732,138 was 48.12 μM for 48 h. Maximum inhibition was observed when the drug was present at a concentration of 100 μM during the culture periods. After the first doubling time, a strong decrease in the cell numbers of the cell line studied was found at intermediate concentrations and no remaining living cells were observed at the maximum concentration. A lower inhibition of growth of the cell line was observed in the presence of low doses of L-732,138 for the GAMG cell line. Figure 3 also show that the standard deviations for the cell line studied were small, pointing to total agreement among the values obtained at the three times the experiments were carried out.

Treatment with L-732,138 at 20 μM partially inhibited the growth of the GAMG cell line (Figure 3). In order to explore whether the NK1 receptor antagonist L-732,138 inhibited cell proliferation via an interaction with its own receptor, we used the specific NK1 receptor agonist SP in competition experiments. Thus, the cellular concentration at 20 μM of L-732,138 and 50 nM of SP was higher (95.08%) than that observed with L-732,138 alone (20 μM) (84.05%). That is, an increase in the cellular concentration (11.03%) was observed in the GAMG cell line treated with both substance P and L-732,138 with respect to the value found when the antagonist was administered alone (Figure 4). These results indicate that L-732,138 blocks SP mitogen stimulation, since L-732,138-induced growth inhibition was partially reversed by the administration of a nanomolar dose of exogenous SP. Finally, there were no significant differences between the control and the control-DMSO groups (data not shown).

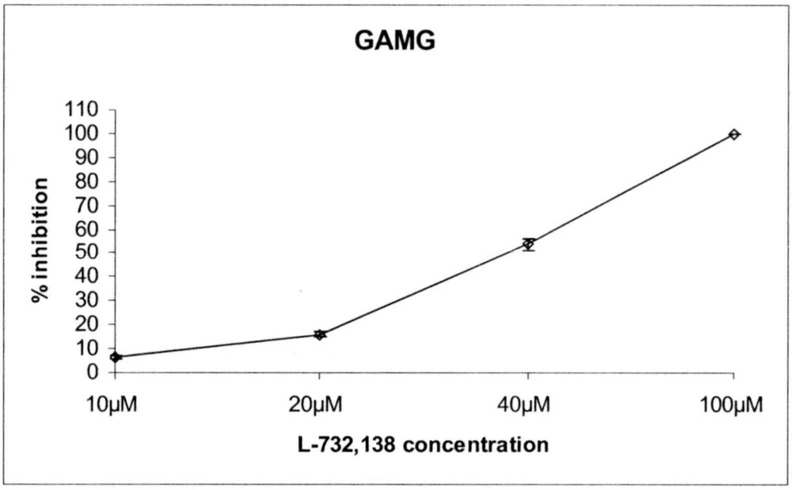

Figure 3. Percentage of growth inhibition of GAMG cells at 48 h in *in vitro* cultures following the addition of increasing concentrations (10, 20, 40 and 100 µM) of L-732,138. The percentage of inhibition for the first doubling time of incubation is plotted on a linear graph. Values are means ± SD (bars).

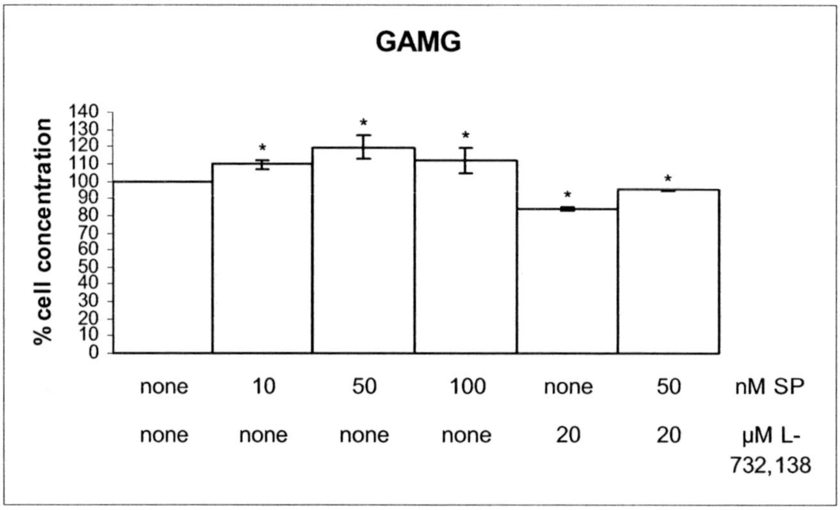

Figure 4. Induction of cell proliferation of GAMG cells by SP at several nanomolar concentrations (10, 50 and 100 nM). The NK1 receptor antagonist L-732,138 was added (20 µM) in the presence (50 nM) or absence (none) of SP for 48 h. In both cases, L-732,138 inhibited GAMG cell proliferation. Using Student's *t*-test, a significant difference between each group (10-none, 50-none, 100-none, none-20, 50-20) and the control group (none-none) was found. Level of significance: * $p \leq 0.01$.

One of the aims of this study was to demonstrate, using a MTS colorimetric method to evaluate cell viability, whether or not the NK1 receptor antagonist L-732,138 exerts an antitumoural action on GAMG glioma cells. Here, we observed that such action occurs through a specific action on the NK1 receptor. Using the non-peptide NK1 receptor antagonist L-732,138, we observed for the first time a potent growth inhibition in the GAMG human cancer cell line. As reported, it has recently been described that the selective non-peptide NK1 receptor antagonist L-733,060 produces a potent growth inhibition in GAMG human cancer cell lines (Muñoz et al., 2004a, 2005a). On comparing the results L-732,138 with L-733,060, we found that the concentration required for a 50% reduction in optical density (IC_{50}) observed in the controls treated with L-732,138 was 48.12 μM for 48 h (see Figure 3), whereas the IC_{50} found for L-733,060 was 21.3 μM (Muñoz et al., 2004a). Thus, we observed a lower antitumoural action of L-732,138 (L-733,060 is two/four-fold more potent that L-732,138). This action could be related with the affinity for the NK1 receptor: 0.8 nM for L-733,060 and 2.3 nM for L-732,138. Thus, at the same concentration used (20 μM), L-733,060 induced a 34.87% of inhibition of the GAMG cells (Muñoz el al., 2004a), whereas L-732,138 only induced a 15% (see Figure 3). In addition, maximun inhibition was observed when L-733,060, at a concentration of 25 μM, was present in the cultures of GAMG cells (Muñoz et al., 2004a). However, the maximun inhibition was observed, after using the NK1 receptor antagonist L-732,138, when a dose of 100 μM was used (see Figure 3). In this case, L-733,060 is four-fold more potent that L-732,138.

Antitumoural Action of NK1 Receptor Antagonists

We have recently demonstrated that L-733,060 displays antitumoural activity against the human SKN-BE(2) neuroblastoma, GAMG glioma, COLO 679, COLO 858, MEL HO melanoma and WERI-Rb-1 and Y-79 retinoblastoma cell lines (Muñoz et al., 2004a, b, 2005a, b), and here we report the antitumoural action of L-732,138 on human GAMG glioma cell line.

Moreover, it has been demonstrated that L-733,060 inhibits the metastatic progression of NK1 receptor-expressed cancer cells and that this NK1 receptor antagonist binds specifically to the human NK1 receptor (Lang et al., 2004). This is in agreement with our results, since in the competition experiments carried out here, exogenous SP cell proliferation was partially reversed by the administration of L-732,138. This indicates that the action on the human neuroblastoma SKN-BE(2) cell line due to the NK1 receptor antagonist L-733,060 (Muñoz et al., 2005a), on the human WERI-Rb-1 and Y-79 retinoblastoma cell lines (Muñoz et al., 2005b) and on the human glioma GAMG cell line by L-733,060 and L-732,138 is related to the ability of these antagonists to block the NK1 receptors expressed by these cell lines (Muñoz et al., 2005a). The growth inhibition of these human cancer cell types using the NK1 receptor antagonists L-733,060/L-732,138 is in agreement with the findings of other studies, in which the use of SP antagonists other than L-733,060/L-732,138 inhibited the growth of both small cell lung cancer and the glioma U373 MG cell line (Woll and Rozengurt, 1988; Langdon et al., 1992; Reeve and Bleehen, 1994; Seckl et al., 1997; Palma et al., 2000).

Currently, we do not know whether the cell death observed in the glioma, neuroblastoma, melanoma and retinoblastoma cell lines (Muñoz et al., 2004a, b, 2005a, b) after treatment with NK1 receptor antagonists would be due to a general toxic effect of L-733,060/L-732,138 or to some specific action of theses substances. Despite this, there are data suggesting the second possibility, since in our competition experiments exogenous SP cell proliferation was partially reversed by administration of L-732,138, as well as by L-733,060 (Muñoz et al., 2005a, b). In addition, it has been described that L-733,060 inhibits the metastatic progression of NK1 receptor-expressing cancer cells (Lang et al., 2004) and that L-733,060 has been successfully used in preclinical assays (at 10-20 mg/kg doses (approximately 30-60 μM)) as anxiolytic and antiinflammatory agents (Bang et al., 2003; Varty et al., 2003). In this sense, it has been reported that L-733,060 dose-dependently protects mice from D-galactosamine/bacterial lipopolysaccharide-induced inflammatory liver injury (edema formation, necrosis…) (Bang et al., 2003). Moreover, the specific binding of L-733,060 to the NK1 receptor has been demonstrated in human breast carcinoma (Lang et al., 2004). In addition, it seems that the antitumoural activity of NK1 receptor antagonists is a specific action and no a general toxic effect for the following reasons: glioma tumour cells express the NK1 receptor (Muñoz et al., 2005a); SP preferentially binds to the NK1 receptor and induces mitogenesis (Muñoz et al., 2005a); and the antitumoural action of the L-732,138/L-733,060 NK1 receptor antagonists is dose-dependent (Muñoz et al., 2004a, 2005a). Moreover, the NK1 receptor antagonists L-733,060 and L- 732,138 are designer molecules that bind specifically to this receptor, with a Ki value of 0.8 nM in the case of L-733,060 and of 2.3 nM for and L- 732,138. Thus, the very structurally different molecules piperidine (L-733,060) and L-tryptophan (L-732,138) have the same antitumoural action and only have in common their specificity for the NK1 receptor. However, on comparing the results obtained with L-732,138 and those with L-733,060 we observed a lower antitumoural action of L-732,138 (L-733,060 is two/four-fold more potent than L-732,138), this action could be related with the affinity for NK1 receptor (0.8 nM for L-733,060 and 2.3 nM for L-732,138). These data suggest that the action of both NK1 receptor antagonists (L-732,138/L-733,060) is antitumoural-specific through the target NK1 receptor (Muñoz et al., 2005a) and that the antitumoural action on cancer cell lines (e.g., glioma, retinoblastoma, neuroblastoma, melanona) by the NK1 receptor antagonists L-733,060 and L-732,138 is probably related to the ability of these antagonists to block the NK1 receptors in such tumours.

The blockade of NK1 receptors in the human SKN-BE neuroblastoma, WERI-Rb-1 and Y-79 retinoblastoma and GAMG glioma cell lines by L-733,060/L-732,138 could inhibit both DNA synthesis and cell proliferation through the mitogen-activated protein kinase (MAPK) pathway (see Luo et al., 1996). L-733,060/L-732,138 could induce growth inhibition by apoptosis, as has been reported previously for in vitro lung cancer cell lines (Reeve and Bleehen, 1994). In this sense, it is known that an SP antagonist (other than L-733,060 or L-732,138) induces apoptosis in lung cancer and causes a concentration-dependent loss of cell viability (Reeve and Bleehen, 1994), as we observed using L-733,060/L-732,138, since the antitumoural activity of L-733,060/L-732,138 reported here was dose-dependent. In addition, it has been described that antiproliferative activity and the induction of apoptosis is observed in vitro in a colon carcinoma cell line (El-Salhy and Starefeldt, 2003), and that in human SH-SY5Y neuroblastoma cells transfected with the galanin receptor subtype GalR2, the activation of the receptor upon galanin treatment completely inhibits cell proliferation and induced apoptosis (Berger et al., 2004). In this latter case, it is the peptide itself (galanin) that produces apoptosis, instead of a galanin receptor antagonist. This also means that the development of galanin agonists could be the basis of future clinical diagnosis and treatment of tumours with high levels of galanin receptor expression like gliomas.

In sum, these data therefore suggest that the antiproliferative action of the NK1 receptor antagonist L-733,060/L-732,138 could involve a signal transduction pathway for apoptosis, after the antagonist has been bound to the NK1 receptors located in the SKH-BE(2), WERI-Rb-1, Y-79 and GAMG cell lines. For gliomas, penetration of the blood-brain barrier by NK1 receptor antagonists might be possible since the barrier is frequently disturbed in glial tumours. However, further studies in this field are necessary to know whether the cell death observed here when the GAMG glioma cell line was treated with L-732,138 would be due to a general toxic effect or to some specific action associated with the ability of this antagonist to block NK1 receptors.

Our results concerning the L-732,138 NK1 receptor antagonist on the GAMG cancer cell line are in agreement with previous findings showing that L-733,060 has antitumoural activity against human cancer cell lines such as neuroblastoma, glioma, retinoblastoma, and melanoma (Muñoz et al., 2004a, b, 2005a, b). It should be noted that in cell lines as different as human neuroblastoma, glioma, retinoblastoma and melanoma the same NK1 receptor antagonist (L-733,060) elicits growth inhibition. This observation suggests the possibility of a common mechanism for cancer cell proliferation mediated by SP and NK1 receptors. Were this the case, it would mean that NK1 receptor antagonists (e.g., L-733,060) could inhibit a large number of tumour cell types in which both SP and NK1 receptors are expressed (Tarkkanen et al., 1983; Lee et al., 1989; Khare et al., 1998; Singh et al., 2000; Friess et al., 2003; Lang et al., 2004), and that they could be candidates as broad-spectrum antineoplastic drugs. In the future, this broad-spectrum action should be also investigated for the NK1 receptor antagonist L-732,138, since in the present work we have demonstrated that this antagonist acts as an antitumoural agent on the GAMG glioma cell line.

Substance P, Inflammation, Pain and Cancer

Several lines of evidence indicate that SP plays a role in regulating neurogenic inflammation and immune responses in both peripheral tissues and in the central nervous system, as we as in pain (see Mantyh, 1991; Harrison and Geppetti, 2001). Thus, the NK1 receptor antagonist L-733,060 has been used as antiinflammatory (Bang et al., 2003) or analgesic (Rupniak et al., 1996) agent. It is known that SP is a potent vasodilator in several peripheral tissues; that terminals containing SP are located close to blood vessels; that the release of SP in peripheral tissues reproduces many of the physiological changes seen in acute inflammation (plasma extravasation...), and that a dramatic up-regulation in the expression of NK1 receptors has been reported during painful chronic conditions (Chahl and Ladda, 1976; Lembeck and Holzer, 1979; Furness et al., 1982; Lundberg et al., 1984).

SP/NK1 receptors can modulate the immune function from sensory nerve/neurogenic inflammation. Moreover, it is known that activation of the SP/NK1 receptor system produces alterations in the humoural (Pascual et al., 1991) and cellular, normal (Feistritzer et al., 2003; Lieb et al., 1997), and tumoural (Luo et al., 1996; Muñoz et al., 2004b) immune response. In this sense, it has been reported that tachykinins are capable of modifying the response of a variety of inflammatory cells, including mast cells, granulocytes, lymphocytes and monocytes and macrophages, and that oedema formation is induced by lower concentrations of SP and is blocked by NK1 receptor antagonists (Walsh et al., 1995). Finally, SP regulation of immune cell function could originate not only from neuronal sources (sensory nerves, neurogenic inflammation), but also from non-neuronal elements, such as eosinophils and macrophages, the expression of both SP and NK1 receptors being up-regulated during inflammation (Weinstock et al., 1988; Cook et al., 1994).

Moreover, it has been described that the number of binding sites for SP, but not for other tachykinins (neurokinin A or B), undergoes huge increases in small arterioles and lymph nodes in human surgical colon samples from patients with inflammatory bowel disease, in comparison with the results found from colon tissue obtained from normal patients (Mantyh, 1991). In other words, the dramatic up-regulation of SP binding sites appears to be restricted to cells involved in mediating the inflammatory (small arterioles) and immune response (lymph nodes) (Mantyh, 1991). In addition, an increase in the levels of SP has been described during intestinal inflammation, and a significant correlation between the degree of inflammation and the clinical status of the disease has been indicated (Keranen et al., 1996a, b). These observations indicate that local release of SP (e. g., in lymph nodes) might be a factor contributing to the immune disorder underlying chronic inflammatory bowel diseases, since in addition the presence of specific SP receptors on human peripheral blood T lymphocytes has been demonstrated (Payan et al., 1984).

In the central nervous system, after transection of the optic nerve an up-regulation of SP binding sites has been observed in astrocytes (Mantyh, 1991), and it has been demonstrated, in vitro, that glia are potential targets for a variety of substances (including the SP) (Muñoz et al., 2004a, 2005a). Thus, by analogy with the inflammatory and immune responses that occur in response to injury in peripheral tissues (Mantyh, 1991), peptides may also regulate glial mitogenesis and the glial response to injury to the central nervous system (see Muñoz et al., 2005a).

Thus, neuroimmune mechanisms are relevant for the perception, maintenance, and perpetuation mechanisms of chronic inflammatory pain. It has been demonstrated that SP-immunoreactive fibers sprout into follicular and nonfollicular accumulations of lymphocytes (Weihe et al., 1991). A disturbed neuroimmune dialogue could well initiate and sustain pain, and there may even be a psycho-neuroimmune-endocrine link. It may be worthwhile to develop drugs for the therapy of pain that normalize disturbed neuroimmune cross-talk.

It is also important to note that in the vast majority of tumours investigated, NK1 receptors have been found in intratumoural and peritumoural blood vessels (Hennig et al., 1995) and that NK1 receptors were highly expressed in blood vessels not only within the tumour mass but also in the peritumoural tissue of pancreatic cancer (Friess et al., 2003).

All these observations suggest that chronic inflammation and pain could produce cancer through the SP/NK1 receptor system, which is up-regulated in the process of chronic inflammation, since it has been demonstrated that SP stimulates mitogenesis (Muñoz et al., 2004b, 2005a, b) and that NK1 receptor expression is increased in cancer cell lines in comparison with normal controls (Friess et al., 2003). In addition, the growth of the tumoural mass, peritumoural infiltration and metastasis could be regulated by the SP/NK1 receptor overexpressed in tumoural cells and in the tumoural and peritumoural tissue (inflammatory cells, fibroblasts, blood vessels, nerves, ganglia, islet) (Friess et al., 2003). Accordingly, treatment with NK1 receptor antagonists could be useful not only for the two above alterations (inflammation and pain), but also for the treatment of tumour cells.

Substance P, Psychiatric Disorders and Cancer: Possible Relationship between the Progression of Cancer and Cerebral Mechanisms

Depression and cancer commonly co-occur. The prevalence of depression among cancer patients increases with disease severity and symptoms such as pain and fatigue. The literature on depression as a predictor of cancer incidence is mixed, although chronic and severe depression may be associated with elevated cancer risk. There is divided but stronger evidence that depression predicts cancer progression and mortality. Moreover, there is evidence that providing psychosocial support reduces depression, anxiety, and pain, and may increase survival time with cancer. Thus, there is evidence of a bi-directional relationship between cancer and depression, offering new opportunities for therapeutic intervention (see Spiegel and Giese-Davis, 2003). In this sense, there are evidences that suggest that factors related to life-style, exposure to various forms of stressors, are associated with mammary tumourgenesis. The possible role of life-style factors in breast cancer is important in light of the fact that mortality to this disease is increasing in most countries and that development of curative therapies for breast cancer has not been forthcoming. The crucial factor affecting tumour growth is the interaction among stress, an individual's personality, and available psychosocial support, and the effect of this interaction on an individual's ability to cope with stress (see Hilakivi-Clarke et al., 1994; Okamura et al., 2005). These data suggest that psychological factors are involved in the development and progression of cancer (Hilakivi-Clarke et al., 1994).

It has been reported that psychotropic drugs modify the expression of the genes encoding the synthesis of tachykinins and the expression of NK1 receptors in selected brain areas (Sivam et al., 1989; Humpel et al., 1990; Shibata et al., 1990). In this sense, chronic treatment with antidepressant drugs produce a decrease in the concentrations of SP in several areas of the central nervous system (striatum, substantia nigra, amygdala...). These findings suggest that a reduction in SP levels in certain brain regions could contribute to a common therapeutic effect of the antidepressant drugs in affective disorders (Shirayama et al., 1996).

In addition to the involvement of SP in depression, the NK1 receptor antagonist L-733,060 has been used as an antidepressive agent (Kramer et al., 1998; Varty et al., 2003) and it has been demonstrated that this antagonist has antitumoural activity against human glioma GAMG and retinoblastoma WERI-Rb-1 and Y-79 cell lines (Muñoz et al., 2004b, 2005b).

Moreover, it is known that the NK1 antagonist Aprepitant (MK-869), an agent structurally unrelated to L-733,060 with antidepressant activity, is as efficient as the antidepressant drug paroxetine in the treatment of depression. The above-mentioned NK1 antagonist is well tolerated and no statistically significant difference in the frequency of adverse events compared to placebo was observed.

SP and NK1 receptors are present in the limbic system, including the hypothalamus and the amygdala. In addition, SP may be involved in the integration of emotional responses to stress, suggesting the possibility that the pathogenesis of depression could be due to an alteration of the SP/NK1 receptor system (Kramer et al., 1998). In fact, in depression an increase in the production of SP has been observed (Kramer et al., 1998).

These data suggest that depression could induce tumour cell proliferation by activating the SP/NK1 receptor system and that treatment with NK1 receptor antagonists could be useful not only for the depression, but also for the treatment of tumour cells. Moreover, all the above data indicate that emotional behaviour (e.g., depression…) (Fehder, 1999; De Vane, 2001), cancer and metastases (Lang et al., 2004) might be related through alterations in the SP/NK1 receptor system. Accordingly, through this system, there could be an interrelationship between the progression of cancer and cerebral mechanisms. The NK1 receptor expressed in the the limbic system are similar to the NK1 receptor expressed on the human tumour cell lines. Moreover, the neuropeptide SP after binding to NK1 receptors located in the limbic system produces anxiety and depression. SP, after binding to the NK1 receptor of the human cell tumour, induces cell proliferation. Therefore, the NK1 receptor antagonists in the limbic system have antidepressant and anxiolytic actions, while the NK1 receptor antagonists in human tumour cell lines have antitumoural action.

Possible Clinical Implications of NK1 Receptor Antagonists

Currently, the antitumoural agents used in clinical practice – the so-called cytostatic drugs - are compounds that show a very low safety profile, and secondary and even very severe side effects and seen (anaemia, leukopenia…). These clinical effects are due to the fact that the drugs are not specific to tumour cells and hence the research accent has always been on the search for a drug with the same or greater antitumoural potential but with fewer side effects. This could only be achieved if the drug were specific to tumour cells.

The action of NK1 receptor antagonists is dose-dependent, and depending on the concentration has more positive effects, at low doses act on NK1 receptos of the brain stem located in the glosopharyngeal nucleus, with an antiemetic action in situations of untractable vomiting by cytostatics. If the dose is raised, the drugs acts on the NK1 receptors at central level in the limbic system (amygdala, hypothalamus, basal nuclei, areas related to emotional behaviour), producing an antidepressive and anxiolytic action. At higher doses, they act on brain areas as a central analgesic. Higher doses still produce an anti-inflammatory action. And similar or slightly higher doses, depending on the tumour in question and its stage, elicit antitumoural activity (inhibition of cellular proliferation, inhibition of the production of metastases, inhibition of peritumour inflammatory reaction and angiogenesis). When used at the highest doses, the NK1 receptor antagonists produce all the positive pharmacological effects described above. This, together with the fact that they are specific to the NK1 receptor and that they are selective to tumour cells (these cells express more NK1 receptors than the non tumoural cells), their action is long-lasting (they are not hydrolysed by peptidases), they can be administered orally, they cross the blood-brain barrier and exert a potent antitumoural action even in melanoma metastases (Muñoz et al., 2004), means that the NK1 receptor antagonists are a promising group of agents for the control and treatment of tumours of the central nervous system.

The possible clinical implications of NK1 receptor antagonists in addition to the inhibition of the growth of tumour cells could be numerous. Thus, the antagonist could be used in movement disorders related to antipsychotic therapy, urinary incontinence, asthma, bronchitis, cough, rhinitis, inflammatory and allergic skin reactions, psoriasis, arthritis, inflammatory bowel disease, colitis, diarrhoea, cystitis and migraine (see Quartara and Maggi, 1998).

Future Research on NK1 Receptor Antagonists

In light of the above nine previous sections, it is clear that there is much to be done if we are to elucidate the role of NK1 receptor antagonists in brain tumours. It is expected that in the near future newer and more effective anticancer drugs (e.g., non-peptide NK1 receptor antagonists) will become available for treatment of tumours of the nervous system . The following points should be addressed in the future in order to increase our knowledge of NK1 receptor antagonists:

1. Determine whether the antiproliferative action of the NK1 receptor antagonists L-732,138 and L-733,060 on cancer cell lines of the human central nervous system (GAMG glioma, retinoblastoma...) might involve a signal transduction pathway for apoptosis.
2. Determine whether the NK1 receptor antagonist L-732,138 could inhibit a large number of tumour cell types in which NK1 receptors are expressed (e.g., retinoblastoma, astrocytoma, neuroblastoma, melanoma...), and, in this sense, investigate the possible antitumoural broad-spectrum action of this antagonist.
3. It would be very interesting to know whether treatment of central nervous system cancer cell lines with the NK1 receptor inhibitors that have been studied in humans (more than thirty compounds) might produce the same growth inhibitory action as was found with L-733,060 or L-732,138 for glioma and retinoblastoma.
4. The functional roles of the different isoforms of the NK1 receptor observed in human GAMG glioma and SKN-BE(2) neuroblastoma cancer cell lines must be investigated.
5. Experiments should be conducted to corroborate the hypothesis that chronic inflammation and pain could produce cancer through the activation of the SP/NK1 receptor system.

6. Demonstrate that depression could induce tumour cell proliferation by activating the SP/NK1 receptor system and that treatment with NK1 receptor antagonists could be useful in depression and for the treatment of tumour cells.
7. Research should address, in experimental animals in vivo, the antiproliferative action of L-732,138 and L-733,060 on central nervous system tumours. It would be interesting to investigate in athymic mice (as in the experiments carried out by Palma et al. (2000) in gliomas) the action of NK1 receptor antagonists (L-732,138/L-733,060 or those used (MEN 11,467, MEN 11,149) by Palma et al. (2000)), but at therapeutic (pharmacological) doses, since the dose used by Palma et al. (2000) was subtherapeutic. Because when Aprepitant (Kramer et al., 1998) was used as an antidepressant in humans the dose was 4.5 mg/kg/day, which is some 10 μM; that is, 10-fold the concentration used by Palma et al. (2000) in mice with gliomas. That author observed that it inhibited in vivo growth, but if higher doses had been used more effective results would probably have been obtained.
8. Using NK1 receptor antagonist agents considered to be drugs (see FDA: Food and Drug Administration), such as Aprepitant, it would be possible to carry out clinical assays in humans and use doses obtained by extrapolating the results collected in vitro against this type of tumour, since in clinical assays it has been observed that these drugs are safe, with side effects like those seen after placebo administration (Kramer et al., 1998).

Conclusion

This study summarizes our findings on the antitumoural action of the NK1 receptor antagonists L-732,138 and L-733,060 on the central nervous system tumoural cell lines (glioma, retinoblastoma) and the results published in previous papers by other authors on the action of the NK1 receptor antagonists, in general, on central nervous system cancer cell lines.

We have demonstrated for the first time in vitro a potent degree of growth inhibition on the human GAMG glioma cell line through use of the non-peptide NK1 receptor antagonist L-732,138, and that the antitumoural action of L-732,138 against this cell line occurs through the NK1 receptors located in this cancer cell line.

In addition, the data presented in this review suggest: 1) that the substance P/NK1 receptor system could play an important role in the development of cancer and metastasis; 2) that substance P may be a universal mitogen in expressed NK1 receptor tumoural cell types; 3) that receptors for several peptides (including the NK1 receptor for SP) have been observed in a broad variety of tumours; 4) that NK1 receptor antagonists act as a broad-spectrum antitumoural agent; 5) that these antagonists could be a promising therapeutic drug for the treatment of human cancer (including central nervous system tumours); 6) and that the NK1 receptor is a new and promising target in the treatment of human cancer cell lines.

Acknowledgements

The authors wish to thank Mr. N. Skinner for stylistic revision of the English text and Mr. Arturo Mangas for technical assistance.

References

Almeida, T; Rojo, J; Nieto, PM. Tachykinins and tachykinin receptor: structure and activity relationships. *Curr Med Chem* 2004; 11, 763-771.

Bang, R; Sass, G; Kiemer, AK; Vollmar, AM; Neuhuber, WL; Tiegs, G. Neurokinin-1 receptor antagonists CP-96,345 and L-733,060 protect mice from cytokine-mediated liver injury. *J Pharmacol Exp Ther* 2003; 305, 31-39.

Berger, A; Lang, R; Moritz, K; Santic, R; Hermann, A; Sperl, W; Kofler, B. Galanin receptor subtype GalR2 mediates apoptosis in SH-SY5Y neuroblastoma cells. *Endocrinology* 2004; 145, 500-507.

Berger, A; Santic, R; Hauser-Kronberger, C; Schilling, FH; Kogner, P; Ratschek, M; Gamper, A; Jones, N; Sperl, W; Kofler, B. Galanin and galanin receptors in human cancers. *Neuropeptides* 2005; 39, 353-359.

Bordey, A; Feltz, P; Trouslard, J. Mobilization of intracellular calcium by substance P in a human astrocytoma cell line (U-373 MG). *Glia* 1994; 11, 277-283.

Bowden, JJ; Garland, AM; Baluk, P; Lefevre, P; Grady, EF; Vigna, SR; Bunnett, NW; McDonald, DM. Direct observation of substance P-induced internalization of NK1 receptors at sites of inflammation. *Proc Natl Acad Sci USA* 1994; 91, 8964-8968.

Burgos, C; Aguirre, JA; Alonso, JR; Coveñas, R. Immunocytochemical study of substance P-like fibres and cell bodies in the cat diencephalon. *J Hirnforsch* 1988; 29, 651-657

Caberlotto, L; Hurd, YL; Murdock, P; Wahlin, JP; Melotto, S; Corsi, M; Carletti, R. Neurokinin 1 receptor and relative abundance of the short and long isoforms in the human brain. *Eur J Neurosci* 2003; 17, 1736-1746.

Cahill, CM; Coderre, TJ. Attenuation of hyperalgesia in a rat model of neuropathic pain after intrathecal pre- or post-treatment with a neurokinin-1 antagonist. *Pain* 2002; 95, 277-285.

Cascieri, MA; MacLeod, AM; Underwood, D; Shiao, LL; Ber, E; Sadowski, S; Yu, H; Merchant, KJ; Swain, CJ; Strader, CD; Fong, TM. Characterization of the interaction of N-acyl-L-tryptophan benzyl ester neurokinin antagonists with the human neurokinin-1 receptor. *J Biol Chem* 1994; 269, 6587-6591.

Chahl, LA; Ladd, RJ. Local oedema and general excitation of cutaneous sensory receptors produced by electrical stimulation of the saphenous nerve in the rat. *Pain* 1976; 2, 25-34.

Cook, GA; Elliott, D; Metwali, A; Blu, AM; Sandor, M; Lynch, R; Weinstock, JV. Molecular evidence that granuloma T lymphocytes in murine *Schistosomiasis mansoni* express an authentic SP (NK1) receptor. *J Immunology* 1994; 152, 1830-1835.

Cuello, AC; Kanazawa, I. The distribution of substance P immunoreactive fibres in the rat central nervous system. *J Comp Neurol* 1978; 178, 129-156.

Cyr, C; South, V; Saltzman, A; Felder, S; Ricca, GA; Jaye, M; Huebner, K; Kagan, J; Croce, CM; Schlessinger, J; Kris, RM. Cloning, expression of the human substance K receptor, and analysis of its role in mitogenesis. *Ann NY Acad Sci* 1991; 632, 426-427.

Dam, TV; Quirion, R. Pharmacological characterization and autoradiographic characterization of substance P receptors in guinea-pig brain. *Peptides* 1986; 7, 855-864.

Danks, JA; Rothman, RB; Cascieri, MA; Chicchi, GG; Liang, T; Herkenham, M. A comparative autoradiographic study of the distributions of substance P and eledoisin binding sites in rat brain. *Brain Res* 1986; 385, 273-281.

De Vane, CL. Substance P: a new era, a new role. *Pharmacotherapy* 2001; 21, 1061-1069.

Diemunsch, P; Grelot, L. Potential of substance P antagonists as antiemetics. *Drugs* 2000; 60, 533-546.

El-Salhy, M; Starefeldt, A. Direct effects of octreotide, galanin and serotonin on human colon cancer cells. *Oncol Rep* 2003; 10, 1723-1728.

Eistetter, HR; Mills, A; Brewster, R; Alouani, S; Rambosson, C; Kawashima, E. Functional characterization of neurokinin-1 receptors on human U373MG astrocytoma cells. *Glia* 1992; 6, 89-95.

Fehder, WP. Alterations in immune response associated with anxiety in surgical patients. *CNRA* 1999; 10, 124-129.

Feistritzer, C; Clausen, J; Sturn, DH; Djanani, A; Gunsilius, E; Wiedermann, CJ; Kahler, CM. Natural killer cell functions mediated by the neuropeptide substance P. *Regul Pep* 2003; 116, 119-126.

Fine, HF. The basis for current recomemmedations for malignant gliomas. *J Neurooncolol* 1994 ; 20, 111-120.

Folkers, K; Feng, D; Asano, N; Hakanson, R; Weisenfeld-Hallin, Z; Leander, S. Spantide II, an effective tachykinin antagonist having high potency and negligible neurotoxicity. *Proc Natl Acad Sci USA* 1990; 87, 4833-4835.

Fowler, CJ; Brannstrom, G. Substance P enhances forskolin-stimulated cyclic AMP production in human UC11MG astrocytoma cells. *Methods Find Exp Clin Pharmacol* 1994; 16, 21-28.

Friess, H ; Zhu, Z ; Liard, V ; Shi, X; Shrikhande, SV; Wang, L; Lieb, K; Korc, M; Palma, C; Zimmermann, A; Reubi, JC; Buchler, MW. Neurokinin-1 receptor expression and its potential effects on tumor growth in human pancreatic cancer. *Lab Invest* 2003; 83, 731-742.

Furness, J; Papka, RE; Della, NG; Costa, M; Eskay, RL. Substance P-like immunoreactivity in nerves associated with the vascular system of guinea-pigs. *Neuroscience* 1982; 7, 447-459.

García, M; Sakamoto, K; Shigekawa, M; Nakanishi, S; Ito, S. Multiple mechanisms of arachidonic acid release in chinese hamster ovary cells transfected with cDNA of SP receptor. *Biochem Pharmacol* 1994; 48, 1735-1741.

Garlan, AM; Grady, EF; Payan, DG; Vigna, SR; Bunnett, NW. Agonist induced internalization of the substance P (NK1) receptor expressed in epithelial cells. *Biochem J* 1994; 303, 177-186.

Giardina, GAM; Gagliardi, S; Martinelli, M. Antagonists at the neurokinin receptors-Recent patent literature. *Drugs* 2003; 6, 758-772.

Globus, M; Smith, MJ; Vethamany-Globus, S. Evidence supporting a mitogenic role for substance P in amphibian limb regeneration. *Ann NY Acad Sci* 1991; 632, 396-399.

Goso, C; Potier, E; Manzini, S; Szallasi, A.Comparison of tachykinin NK1 receptors in human IM9 and U373 MG cells, using antagonist (FK888, (+/-)-CP-96,345, and RP 67580) binding. *Eur J Pharmacol* 1994; 254, 221-227.

Grady, EF; Garland, AM; Gamp, PD; Lovett, M; Payan, DG; Bunnett, NW. Delineation of the endocytic pathway of substance P and its seven transmembrane domains NK1 receptor. *Mol Biol Cell* 1995; 6, 509-524.

Hammond, PJ; Smith, DM; Akinsanya, KO; Mufti, WA; Wynick, D; Bloom, SR. Signalling patways mediating secretory and mitogenic responses to galanin and pituitary adenylate cyclase-activating polypeptide in the 235-1 clonal rat lactotroph cell line. *J Neuroendocrinol* 1996; 8, 457-464.

Harrison, S; Geppetti, P. Substance P. *Int J Biochem Cell Biol* 2001; 33, 555-576.

Harrison, T; Williams, BJ; Swain, CJ; Ball, RG. Piperidine-ether based hNK1 antagonists 1: determination of the relative and absolute stereochemical requirements. *Biomed Chem Lett* 1994; 4, 2545-2550.

Hennig, IM; Laissue, JA; Horisberger, U; Reubi, JC. Substance-P receptors in human primary neoplasms: tumoral and vascular localization. *Int J Cancer* 1995; 61, 786-792.

Hershey, AD; Polenzani, L; Woodward, RM; Miledi, R; Krause, JE. Molecular and genetic characterization, functional expression, and mRNA expression patterns of a rat substance P receptor. *Ann NY Acad Sci* 1991; 632, 63-78.

Hilakivi-Clarke, L; Rowland, J; Clarke, R; Lippman, ME. Psychosocial factors in the development and progression of breast cancer. *Breast Cancer Res Treat* 1994; 29, 141-160.

Hökfelt, T; Pernow, B; Wahren, J. Substance P: a pioneer amongst neuropeptides. *J Intern Med* 2001; 249, 27-40.

Hökfelt, T; Pernow, B; Nilsson, G; Wetterberg, L; Goldstein, M; Jeffcoate, SL. Dense plexus of substance P-immunoreactive nerve terminals in eminentia medialis of the primate hypothalamus. *Proc Natl Acad Sci USA* 1978; 74, 1013-1015.

Hossen, MA; Fujii, Y; Sugimoto, Y; Kayasuga, R; Kamei, C. Histamine H3 receptors regulate vascular permeability changes in the skin of mast cell-deficient mice. *Int Immunopharmacol,* 2003; 3, 1563-1568

Humpel, C; Knaus, GA; Auer, B; Knaus, HG; Haring, C; Theodorsson, E; Saria, A. Effects of haloperidol and clozapine on preprotachykinin mRNA tachykinin tissue level release and NK1 receptors in the striatonigral system. *Synapse* 1990; 6, 1-9.

Johnson, CL; Johnson, CG. Substance P regulation of glutamate and cystine transport in human astrocytoma cells. *Receptor Channel* 1993; 1, 53-59.

Johnson, CL; Johnson, CG; Stauderman, KA, Buck, SH. Characterization of substance P receptors in human astrocytoma cells. *Ann NY Acad Sci* 1991; 632, 410-412.

Kaneko, A; Suzuki, S. Eye-preservation treatment of retinoblastoma with vitreous seeding. *Jpn J Clin Oncol* 2003; 33, 601-617.

Keranen, U; Jarvinen, H; Kiviluoto, T; Kivilaakso, E; Soinila, S. Substance P and VIP-immunoreactive innervation in normal and inflamed pouches after restorative proctocolectomy for ulcerative colitis. *Dig Dis Sci* 1996a; 41, 1658-1664.

Keranen, U; Jarvinen, H; Karkkaine, P; Kiviluoto, T; Kivilaakso, E; Soinila, S. Substance P – an underlying factor for pouchitis?. Prospective study of substance P and VIP-immunoreactive innervation and mast cells. *Dig Dis Sci* 1996b; 41, 1665-1671.

Khare, VK; Albino, AP; Reed, JA. The neuropeptide/mast cell secretagogue substance P is expressed in cutaneus melanocytic lesions. *J Cutan Pathol* 1998; 25, 2-10.

Kleihues, P; Cavanee, WK. World Health Organization classification of tumours: tumours of the nervous system. *Pathology and genetics*. First edition. Lyon: IRAC Press; 2000.

Koglin, N; Beck-Sickinger, AG. Novel modified and radiolabelled neuropeptide Y analogues to study Y-receptor subtypes. *Neuropeptides* 2004; 38, 153-161.

Kramer, MS; Cutler, N; Feighner, J; Shrivastava, R; Carman, J; Sramek, JJ; Reines, SA; Liu, G; Snavely, D; Wyatt-knowles, E; Halle, JJ; Mills, SG; MacCoss, M; Swain, CJ; Harrison, T; Hill, RG; Hefti, F; Scolnick, EM; Cascieri, MA; Chicchi, GG; Sadowski, S; Williams, AR; Hewson, L; Smith, D; Carlsson, EJ; Hargreaves, RJ; Rupniak, NM. Distinct mechanism for antidepressant activity by blockade of central substance P receptors. *Science* 1998; 281, 1640-1645.

Lackie, JM; Dow, JAT. *The dictionary of cell biology*. Second edition. London: Academic Press; 1995.

Lang, K; Drell, TL; Lindecke, A; Niggemann, B; Kaltschmidt, C; Zaenker, KS; Entschladen, F. Induction of a metastatogenic tumor cell type by neurotransmitters and its pharmacological inhibition by established drugs. *Int J Cancer* 2004; 112, 231-238.

Langdon, S; Sethi, T; Richie, A; Muir, M; Smyth, J; Rozengurt, E. Broad spectrum neuropeptide antagonists inhibit the growth of small cell lung cancer in vivo. *Cancer Res* 1992; 52, 4554-4557.

Lee, CM; Campbell, NJ; Williams, BJ; Iversen, LL. Molecular characterization of a functional cDNA for rat receptor. *Eur J Pharmacol* 1986; 130, 209-217.

Lee, CM; Kum, W; Cockram, CS; Teoh, R; Young, JD. Functional substance P receptors on a human astrocytoma cell line (U-373 MG). *Brain Res* 1989; 488, 328-331.

Lee, CM; Tung, WL; Young, JD. Tachykinin-stimulated inositol phospholipid hydrolysis and taurine release from human astrocytoma cells. *J Neurochem* 1992; 59, 406-414.

Lembeck, F; Holzer, P. Substance P as neurogenic mediator of antidromic vasodilation and neurogenic plasma extravasation. *Naunyn-Schmiedeberg's Arch Pharmacol* 1979; 310, 175-183.

Lieb, K; Fiebich, BL; Berger, M; Bauer, J; Schulze-Osthoff, K. The neuropeptide substance P activates transcription factors NF.kB and kB-dependent gene expression in human astrocytoma cells. *J Immunol* 1997; 159, 4952-4958.

Lotz, M; Carson, DA; Vaughan, JH. Substance P activation of rheumatoid synoviocytes: neural pathway in pathogenesis of arthritis. *Science* 1987; 235, 893-895.

Lundberg, JM; Brodin, E; Hua, X; Saria, A. Vascular permeability changes and smooth muscle contraction in relation to capsaicin-sensitive substance P afferents in the guinea-pig. *Acta Physiol Scand* 1984; 120, 217-227.

Luo, W; Sharif, TR; Sharif, M. Substance P-induced mitogenesis in human astrocytoma cells correlates with activation of the mitogen-activated protein kinase signaling pathway. *Cancer Res* 1996; 56, 4983-4991.

MacDonald, SG; Boyd, ND. Regulation of substance P receptor affinity by guanine nucleotide binding proteins. *J Neurochem* 1989; 53, 264-272.

MacLeod, AM; Merchant, KJ; Brookfield, F; Kelleher, F; Stevenson, G; Owens, AP; Swain, CJ; Cascieri, MA; Sadowski, S; Ber, E; Strader, CD; Fong, TM. Identification of L-tryptophan derivatives with potent and selective antagonist activity at the NK1 receptor. *J Med Chem* 1994; 37, 1269- 1274.

Maeno, H; Kiyama, H; Tohyama, M. Distribution of the substance P (NK1) receptor in the central nervous system. *Mol Brain Res* 1993; 18, 43-58.

Maggi, CA; Patacchini, R; Rovero, P; Giachetti, A. Tachykinin receptors and receptor antagonists. *J Auton Pharmacol* 1993; 13, 958-962.

Mai, JK; Stephens, PH; Hopf, A; Cuello, AC. Substance P in the human brain. *Neuroscience* 1986; 17, 709-739.

Mantyh, PW. Substance P and the inflammatory and immune response. *Ann NY Acad Sci* 1991; 632, 263-271.

Mantyh, PW; Allen, CJ; Ghilardi, JR; Rogers, SD; Mantyh, CR; Liu, H; Basbaum, AI; Vigna, SR; Maggio, JE. Rapid endocytosis of a G protein-coupled receptor: substance P evoked internalization of its receptor in the rat striatum in vivo. *Proc Natl Acad Sci USA*. 1995; 92, 2622-2626.

Maxwell, M; Naber, SP; Wolfe, HJ; Galanopoulos, T; Hedley-Whyte, ET; Black, PM; Antoniades, HN. Coexpression of platelet-derived growth factor (PDGF) and PDGF-receptor genes by primary human astrocytomas may contribute to their development and maintenance. *J Clin Invest* 1990; 86, 131-140.

McGillis, JP; Mitsuhashi, M; Payan, DG. Immunomodulation by tachykinin neuropeptides. *Ann NY Acad Sci* 1990; 594, 85-94.

Medrano, S; Gruenstein, E; Dimlich, RV. Sunstance P receptor on human astrocytoma cells are linked to glycogen breakdown. *Neurosci Lett* 1994; 167, 14-18.

Mitsuhashi, M; Ohashi, Y; Schichijo, S; Christian, C; Sudduth-Klinger, J; Harrowe, G; Payan, DG. Multiple intracellular signalling pathways of the neuropeptide SP receptor. *J Neurosci Res* 1992; 32, 437-443.

Mochizuki-Oda, N; Nakajima, Y; Nakanishi, S; Ito, S. Characterization of the SP receptor-mediated Ca influx in cDNA transfected CHO cells. *J Biol Chem* 1994; 269, 9651-9658.

Muñoz, M; Pérez, A; Coveñas, R; Rosso, M; Castro E. Antitumoural action of L-733,060 on neuroblastoma and glioma cell lines. *Arch Ital Biol* 2004a; 142, 105-112.

Muñoz, M; Pérez, A; Rosso, M; Zamarriego, C; Rosso, R. Antitumoural action of NK1 receptor antagonist L-733,060 on human melanoma cell lines. *Melanoma Res* 2004b; 14, 183-188.

Muñoz, M ; Rosso, M ; Pérez, A ; Coveñas, R ; Rosso, R ; Zamarriego, C ; Piruat, JI. The NK1 receptor is involved in the antitumoural action of L-733,060 and in the mitogenic action of substance P on neuroblastoma and glioma cell lines. *Neuropeptides* 2005a; 39, 427-432.

Muñoz, M ; Rosso, M ; Pérez, A ; Coveñas, R ; Rosso, R ; Zamarriego, C ; Soult, JA ; Montero, I. Antitumoural action of the neurokinin-1- receptor antagonist L-733,060 and mitogenic action of substance P on human retinoblastoma cell lines. *Invest Ophthalmol Vis Sci* 2005b; 46, 2567-2570.

Nakajima, Y; Tsuchida, K; Negishi, M; Ito, S; Nakanishi, S. Direct linkage of three tachykinin receptors to stimulation of both phosphatidylinositol hydrolysis and cAMP cascades in transfected chinese hamster ovary cells. *J Biol Chem* 1992; 267, 2437-2442.

Nakata, Y; Hiraoka, C; Segawa, T. Apparent molecular weight of the substance P binding site in rat brain. *Eur J Pharmacol* 1988; 152, 171-174.

Nakaya, Y; Kaneko, T; Shigemoto, R; Nakanishi, S; Mizuno, N. Immunohistochemical localization of substance P receptor in the central nervous system of the adult rat. *J Comp Neurol* 1994; 347, 249-274.

Nilsson, J; von Euler, AM; Dalsgaard, CJ. Stimulation of connective tissue cell growth by substance P and substance K. *Nature* 1985; 315, 61-63.

Nowicki, M; Miskowiak, B. Comparison of the cell immunophenotype of metastatic and primary foci in stage IV-S neuroblastoma. *Folia Histochem Cytobiol* 2002; 40, 297-303.

Okamura, M; Yamawaki, S; Akechi, T; Taniguchi, K; Uchitomi, Y. Psychiatric disorders following first breast cancer recurrence: prevalence, associated factors and relationship to quality of life. *Jpn J Clin Oncol*, 2005; 35, 302-309.

Organist, ML; Harvey, JP; McGillis, JP; Payan, DG. Processing of the human IM-9 lymphoblast substance P receptor. Biosynthetic and degradation studies using a monoclonal anti-receptor antibody. *Biochem Biophys Res Commun* 1988; 151, 535-541.

Oury-Donat, F; Lefevre, IA; Thurneyssen, O; Gauthier, T; Bordey, A; Feltz, P; Edmonds-Alt, X; Le Fur, G; Soubrie, P. SR 140333, a novel, selective, and potent nonpeptide antagonist of the NK1 tachykinin receptor: characterization on the U373 MG cell line. *J Neurochem* 1994; 62, 1399-1407.

Palma, C; Manzini, S. Substance P induces secretion of immunomodulatory cytokines by human astrocytoma cells. *J Neuroimmunol* 1998; 81, 127-137.

Palma, C; Bigioni, M; Irrissuto, C; Nardelli, F; Maggi, CA; Manzini, S. Anti-tumour activity of tachykinin NK1 receptor antagonists on human glioma U373 MG xenograft. *Br J Cancer* 2000; 82, 480-487.

Palma, C; Nardelli, F; Manzini, S; Maggi, CA. Substance P activates responses correlated with tumour growth in human glioma cells line bearing tachykinin NK1 receptors. *Br J Cancer* 1999; 79, 236-243.

Pascual, DW; Xu-Amano, J; Kiyono H; McGhee, JR; Bost, KL. Substance P acts directly upon cloned B Lymphoma cells to enhace IgA and IgM production. *J Immunol* 1991; 146, 2130-2136.

Payan, DG; Brewster, DR; Goetzl, EJ. Specific stimulation of human T lymphocytes by substance P. *J Immunol* 1983; 131, 1613-1615.

Payan, DG; Brewster, DR; Missirian-Bastian, A; Goetzl, EJ. Substance P recognition of a subset of human T lymphocytes. *J Clin Investigation* 1984; 74, 1532-1539.

Payan, DG; McGillis, JP; Organist, ML. Binding characteristics and affinity labeling of protein constituents of the human IM-9 lymphoblast receptor for substance P . *J Biol Chem* 1986; 261, 14321-14329.

Perentes, E; Herbort, CP; Rubinstein, LJ; Herman, MM; Uffer, S; Donoso, LA; Collins, VP. Immunohistochemical characterization of human retinoblastomas in situ with multiple markers. *Am J Ophthalmol* 1987; 103, 647-658.

Pernow, B. Substance P. *Pharmacol Rev* 1983; 35, 85-141.

Plate, KH; Breier, G; Farrell, CL; Risau, W. Platelet-derived growth factor receptor-beta is induced during tumor development and upregulated during tumor progression in endothelial cells in human gliomas. *Lab Invest* 1992; 67, 529-534.

Quartara, L; Maggi, CA. The tachykinin NK1 receptor. Part I: ligands and mechanisms of cellular activation. *Neuropeptides* 1997; 31, 537-563.

Quartara, L; Maggi, CA. The tachykinin NK1 receptor. Part II: distribution and pathophysiological roles. *Neuropeptides* 1998; 32, 1-49.

Reeve, JG; Bleehen, NM. [D-Arg^{1}-D-Phe^{5}, D-Trp^{7,9}, Leu^{11}] Substance P induces apoptosis in lung cancer cell lines in vitro. *Biochem Bioph Res Com* 1994; 199, 1313-1319.

Regoli, D; Boudon, A; Fauchere, J. Receptors and antagonists for substance P and related peptides. *Pharmacol Rev* 1994; 46, 551-599.

Reid, RC. Vision. In: Zigmond MJ, Bloom FE, Landis SC, Roberts JL, Squire LR. *Fundamental neuroscience*. San Diego. Academic Press; 1999; pp. 821-851.

Reubi, JC. Peptide receptors as molecular targets for cancer diagnosis and therapy. *Endocr Rev* 2003; 24, 389-427.

Rupniak, NM; Carlson, E; Boyce, S; Webb, JK; Hill, RG. Enantioselective inhibition of the formalin paw late phase by the NK1 receptor antagonist L-733,060 in gerbils. *Pain* 1996; 67, 189-195.

Rupniak, NM; Carlson, EC; Harrison, T; Oates, B; Seward, E; Owen, S; de Felipe, C; Hunt, S; Wheeldon, A. Pharmacological blockade or genetic deletion of substance P (NK(1)) receptors attenuates neonatal vocalisation in guinea-pigs and mice. *Neuropharmacology* 2000; 39, 1413-1421.

Saffroy, M; Beaujouan, JC; Torrens, Y; Besseyre, J; Bergstrom, L; Glowinski, J. Localization of tachykinin binding sites (NK1, NK2, NK3 ligands) in the rat brain. *Peptides* 1988; 9, 227-241.

Salo, E; Baguna, T. Stimulation of cellular proliferation and differentiation in the intact and regenerating planarian Dugesia(G) tigrina by the neuropeptide substance P. *J Exp Zool* 1986; 237, 129-135.

Samsam, M; Coveñas, R; Ahangari, R; Yajeya, J; Narváez, JA; Tramu, G. Simultaneous depletion of neurokinin A, substance P and calcitonin gene-related peptide from the caudal trigeminal nucleus of the rat during electrical stimulation of the trigeminal ganglion. *Pain* 2000; 84, 389-395.

Schlegel, U; Moots, PL; Rosenblum, MK; Thaler, HT; Furneaux, HM. Expression of transforming growth factor alpha in human gliomas. *Oncogene* 1990; 5, 1839-1842.

Seabrook, GR; Fong, TM. Thapsigargin blocks the mobilization of intracellular Ca caused by activation of human NK1 (long) receptors expressed in CHO cells. *Neurosci Lett* 1993; 152, 9-12.

Seckl, MJ; Higgins, T; Wildmer, F; Rozengurt, E. [D-Arg^{1}, D-Trp^{5,7,9}, Leu^{11}] Substance P: a novel potent inhibitor of signal transduction and growth in vitro and in vivo in small cell lung cancer cells. *Cancer Res* 1997; 57, 51-54.

Seufferlein, T; Rozengurt, E. Galanin, neurotensin, and phorbol esters rapidly stimulate activation of mitogen-activated protein kinase in small cell lung cancer cells. *Cancer Res* 1996; 56, 5758-5764.

Sharif, TR; Luo, W; Houghron, PJ; Sharif, M. Substance K peptide induces mitogenesis by activating the mitogen-activated protein kinase signalling pathway through the substance P receptor (NK-1 subtype) in human astrocytoma. *Cell Pharmacol* 1996; 3, 441-449.

Shibata, K; Haverstick, DM; Bannon, MJ. Tachykinin gene expression in rat limbic nuclei: modulation by dopamine antagonists. *J Pharmacol Exp Ther* 1990; 255, 388-392.

Shields, CL; Shields, JA. Recent developments in the management of retinoblastoma. *J Pediatr Ophthalmol Strabismus* 1999; 36, 8-18.

Shields, CL; Shields, JA. Diagnosis and management of retinoblastoma. *Cancer Control* 2004; 11, 317-327.

Shirayama, Y; Mitsushio, H; Takashima, M; Ichikawa, H; Takayashi, K. Reduction of substance P after chronic antidepressant treatment in the striatum, substantia nigra and amygdala of the rat. *Brain Res* 1996; 739, 70-78.

Shrestha, P; Yang, L; Liu, B; Namba, M; Takagi, H; Hosaka, M; Mori, M. Neuroblastoma of parotid gland: report of a case and immunohistochemical characteristics. *Eur J Cancer B Oral Oncol* 1994; 30, 356-361.

Singh, D; Joshi, DD; Hameed, M; Qian, J; Gascon, P; Maloof, PB; Mosenthal, A; Rameshwar, P. Increased expression of preprotachykinin-I and neurokinin receptors in human breast cancer cells: implications for bone marrow metastasis. *Proc Natl Acad Sci USA* 2000; 97, 388-393.

Sivam, SP; Krause, JE; Takeuchi, K; Li, S; McGinty, J; Hong, JS. Lithium increases rat striatal β- and γ-preprotachykinin messenger RNAs. *J Pharmacol Exp Ther* 1989; 248, 1297-1301.

Snider, RM; Constantine, JW; Lowwe, IJ. A potent nonpeptide antagonist of the substance P (NK1) receptor. *Science* 1991; 251, 435-437.

Spiegel, D; Giese-Davis, J. Depression and cancer: mechanisms and disease progression. *Biol Psychiatry* 2003; 54, 269-282.

Stockhammer, G; Manley, GT; Johnson, R; Rosenblum, MK; Samid, D; Lieberman, FS. Inhibition of proliferation and induction of differentiation in medulloblastoma- and astrocytoma-derived cell lines with phenylacetate. *J Neurosurg* 1995; 83, 672-681.

Takahashi, JA; Mori, H; Fukumoto, M; Igarashi, K; Jaye, M; Oda, Y; Kikuchi, H; Hatanaka, M. Gene expression of fibroblast growth factors in human gliomas and meningiomas: demonstration of cellular source of basic fibroblast growth factor mRNA and peptide in tumor tissues. *Proc Natl Acad Sci USA* 1990; 87, 5710-5714.

Takeda, Y; Blount, P; Sachais, BS; Hershey, AD; Raddatz, R; Krause, JE. Ligand binding kinetics of substance P and neurokinin A receptors stably expressed in CHO cells and evidence for differential stimulation of inositol 1, 4, 5-triphosphate and camp second messenger responses. *J Neurochem* 1992; 59, 740-745.

Tamboli, A; Podgor, MJ; Horm, JW. The incidence of retinoblastoma in the United States: 1974 through 1985. *Arch Ophthalmol* 1990; 108, 128-132.

Tarkkanen, A; Tervo, T; Tervo, K; Eranko, L; Eranko, O; Cuello, AC. Substance P immunoreactivity in normal human retina and in retinoblastoma. *Ophthalmic Res* 1983; 15, 300-306.

Torrens, Y ; Beaujouan, JC ; Saffroy, M; Glowinski, J; Tence, M. Functional coupling of the NK1 tachykinin receptor to phospholipase D in Chinese hamster ovary cells ans astrocytoma cells. *J Neurochem* 1998; 70, 2091-2098.

Turner, AJ. Endopeptidase-24.11 and neuropeptide metabolism. In: Turner AJ, *Neuropeptides and Their Peptidases*. Chichester: Ellis Horwood; 1987; pp. 183-201.

Unger, T; Rascher, W; Schuster, C; Pavlovitch, R; Schömig, A; Dietz, R; Ganten, D. Central blood pressure effects of substance P and angiotensin II: role of the sympathetic nervous system and vasopressin. *Eur J Pharmacol* 1981; 71, 33-42.

van Ginkel, FW; Pascual, DW. Recognition of neurokinin 1 receptor (NK1-R): an antibody to a peptide sequence from the third extracellular region binds to brain NK1-R. *J Neuroimmunol* 1996; 67, 49-58.

Varty, GB; Cohen-Williams, ME; Hunter, JC. The antidepressant-like effects of neurokinin NK1 receptor antagonists in a gerbil tail suspension test. *Behav Pharmacol* 2003; 14, 87-95.

von Euler, US ; Gaddum, JH. An unidentified depressor substance in certain tissue extracts. *J Physiol* 1931; 72, 74-87.

Walsh, DT; Weg, VB; Williams, TJ; Nourshargh, S. Substance P induced inflammatory responses in guinea-pig skin: the effect of specific NK1 receptor antagonists and the role of endogenous mediators. *Br J Pharmacol* 1995; 114, 1343-1350.

Weihe, E; Nohr, D; Müller, S; Büchler, M; Friess, H; Zentel, H-J. The tachykinin neuroimmune connection in inflammatory pain. *Ann NY Acad Sci* 1991; 632, 283-295.

Weinstock, JV; Blum, A; Walden, J; Walden, T. Eosinophils from granulomas in murine *Schistosomiasis mansoni* produce SP. *J Immunology* 1988; 141, 961-966.

Whitty, CJ; Walker, PD; Goebel, DJ; Poosch, MS; Bannon, MJ. Quantitation, cellular localization and regulation of neurokinin receptor gene expression whithin the rat substantia nigra. *Neuroscience* 1995; 64, 419-425.

Wolf, SS; Moody, TW; Quirion, R; O'Donahue, TL. Biochemical characterization and autoradiographic localization of central SP receptor using [^{125}I] physalaemin. *Brain Res* 1985; 332, 299-307.

Woll, PJ; Rozengurt E. [D-Arg^{1}-D-Phe^{5}, D-Trp^{7,9}, Leu^{11}] Substance P, a potent bombesin antagonist in murine Swiss 3T3 cells, inhibits the growth of human small cell lung cancer cells in vitro. *Proc Natl Acad Sci USA* 1988; 35, 1859-1863.

Wrensch, M; Minn, Y; Chew, T; Bondy, M; Berger, MS. Epidemiology of primary brin tumors: current concepts and review of the literature. *Neuro-oncol* 2002; 4, 278-299.

Ziche, M; Morbidelli, L; Pacini, M; Dolara, P; Maggi, CA. NK1-receptors mediate the proliferative response of human fibroblasts to tachykinins. *Br J Pharmacol* 1990; 100, 11-14.

In: Brain Cancer: Therapy and Surgical Interventions... ISBN 1-59454-974-5
Editor: Andrew V. Yang, pp. 77-111

Chapter IV

Targeted Therapy for Brain Tumors

Stanislaw R. Burzynski
Burzynski Research Institute

Abstract

Therapeutic agents affecting specific targets in cancer cells have begun to occupy an important position in cancer treatment. These treatments, known as targeted therapies, exert their effect via two main mechanisms. One group of these therapeutic agents is monoclonal antibodies which block receptors on the cell surface, deliver anti-neoplastic agents or facilitate the immune response. A second group of agents are small molecules which enter the cell and interrupt signaling pathways necessary for cancerous growth. Several drugs which affect single targets are used successfully for malignancies outside the brain in oncological practice. Imatinib mesylate, gefitinib, erlotinib, bevacizumab, inhibitors of farnesyltransferase and multitargeted agents such as antineoplastons (ANP) are also being used in extensive clinical studies in neuro-oncology. Imatinib, gefitinib and erlotinib do not appear to have antitumor activity in high-grade gliomas as single agents, but may produce a synergistic effect with chemotherapy. ANP shows promising results in phase II studies of high and low grade gliomas, brain stem gliomas and a number of responses in preliminary reports in primitive neuroectodermal tumors, atypical teratoid/rhabdoid tumors and multicentric gliomas. The efficacy of these agents has not yet been confirmed in phase III studies. This chapter reviews the most important molecular targets, mechanisms of action and results of clinical trials of new generation of antineoplastic drugs that selectively destroy neoplastic cells in brain tumors.

Introduction

The idea of developing drugs which are oriented against specific targets is not new and can be traced back to Paul Ehrlich whose 150th birthday anniversary was celebrated in the fall of 2004 [1,2]. The science of medicinal chemistry, which was founded by Ehrlich at the beginning of the 20th century, relied on libraries of synthetic and natural products that were screened in selected types of bioassays. The idea originated from Paul Ehrlich's research on synthetic dyes, which specifically stained targets in microorganisms. In collaboration with Hoechst Farbwerke, Ehrlich's team developed a targeted library of hundreds of compounds. In the fall of 1909, compound No. 606 from his library, named salvarsan, dramatically proved the validity of his idea [1]. A new generation of drugs that recognized specific targets are opening new perspectives for cancer treatment. The drugs which were initially approved for oncological indications were oriented against single specific targets. They raised tremendous hopes and excitement as well as disappointment [3]. The treatment of chronic myelogenous leukemia with imatinib resulted in dramatic responses and durable results in many patients. This is easy to understand since there is a clearly identifiable molecular target for imatinib in Philadelphia chromosome. The drugs which were developed to interrupt signal transduction in the pathways involving the members of the family of human epidermal growth factor receptor (HER) were less successful. The gene for HER2 (*ERBB2*) is amplified in approximately 1/3 of breast cancers. Trastuzumab, which is anti-HER2 antibody, may produce responses up to 35% of patients with marked over-expression of *ERBB2* in cancer cells [4]. Epidermal growth factor receptor (EGFR/ERBB1) inhibitor gefinitib was not as successful. It was approved by the FDA as a third line therapy for non-small-cell lung cancer based on phase II trials [5]. The results of phase III trial of gefitinib, in addition to chemotherapy, were disappointing and did not confirm prior clinical observations [6, 7]. To the contrary, the addition of chemotherapy enhanced responses to trastuzumab and resulted in extension of patients' survival [8].

Primary brain tumors are among the most disappointing diagnoses, both for patients and their physicians. With the exception of a small percentage of patients who have successful total surgery, in the majority of cases the disease will progress and lead to death, despite radiation therapy and chemotherapy [9]. The addition of temozolomide (TMZ) improved short-term results but did not change the final outcome [10, 11]. Further research confirmed that the benefits of TMZ were limited to the minority of patients with methylation of the promoter of 0_6-methylguanine-DNA methyltransferase (MGMT) [12]. Increased angiogenesis in brain tumors raised hopes that antiangiogenic therapy will provide better results. The first antiangiogenic drug approved by FDA-thalidomide was used in phase II trials of glioblastoma multiforme (GBM) and anaplastic astrocytoma (AA). Four different clinical studies using thalidomide as a single agent, and in combination with TMZ, carboplatin and radiation therapy did not provide the proof of efficacy and contributed to serious thromboembolic events [13-17]. It is the expert's opinion that the advancement in treatment of patients with brain tumors has been negligible and a completely new approach is needed for a significant change [9, 18]. The present chapter is trying to answer the question if targeted therapy may improve dismal results of the treatment of brain tumors? The author reviews the most important strategies which resulted in introduction of the agents which can be useful in the treatment of brain tumors. The results of phase II trials are discussed and summarized.

Targeted Therapeutic Agents Used for Treatment of Primary Brain Tumors

The emphasis of research on pharmaceutical agents is centered on drugs effecting pre-selected targets. The last 10 years have seen dynamic expansion of the interest in this area. From approximately 500 molecular targets in 1996, the current therapeutic target database contains over 1200 targets [19]. In the area of neoplastic diseases, the current list includes 392 targets [19]. The therapeutic targets are extensively described in the literature. In this chapter, the attention is concentrated on the agents used in phase II clinical trials for primary brain tumors. Most of these agents affect single targets, including growth factor receptors, signal transduction pathways, G1-S transition, apoptosis, membrane transport or epigenetic changes. (Figure 1) Table 1 lists currently used drugs and their targets.

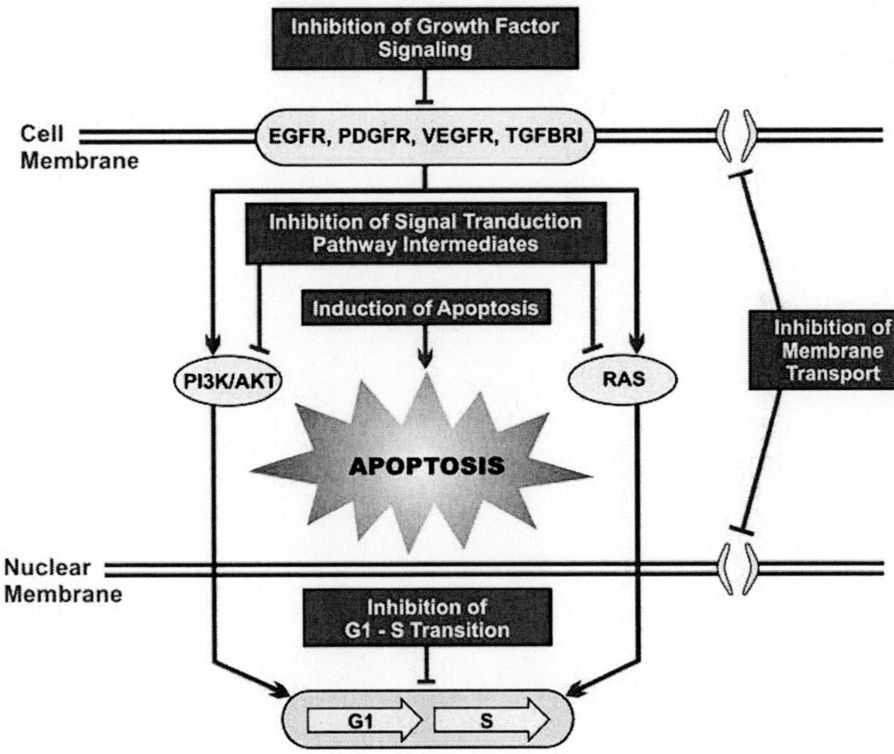

Figure 1. Targets for therapeutic agents used for treatment of primary brain tumors. EGFR, PDGFR, VEGFR, TGFBR1- growth factor receptors, PI3K/AKT, RAS - oncogene proteins, G1-S-phases of cell cycle.

Table 1. Targeted Therapeutic Agents in Clinical Use for Primary Brain Tumors

Agent	Brand Name	Company	Target	Type	Status Brain Tumors	Indication Approved
Generic Name						
Imatinib	Gleevec	Novartis	BCR-ABL	TKI	Phase II	Chronic myelogenous leukemia
Gefitinib	Iressa	Astra Zeneca	EGFR	TKI	Phase II	Advanced non-small cell lung cancer
Erlotinib	Tarceva	Genentech/OSI	EGFR	TKI	Phase II	Non-small cell lung cancer, pancreatic cancer
Lonafarnib	Sarasar	Shering-Plough	RAS	Peptidomimetic	Phase II	
Bevacizumab	Avastin	Genentech	VEGF	Monoclonal antibody	Phase II	Colorectal cancer in combination with 5-fluorouracil
Enzastaurin		Eli Lilly	PKC-β2 (VEGF)	PKC-β2 inhibitor	Phase II	
Temsirolimus (CCI-779)		Wyeth	mTOR	mTOR inhibitor	Phase II	
ANP - A10I	Atengenal	BRI	Multitargeted	DMM	Phase II	
ANP - AS2-1I	Astugenal	BRI	Multitargeted	DMM	Phase II	
ANP - A10	Cengenal	BRI	Multitargeted	DMM	Phase II	
ANP - AS2-1	Fengenal	BRI	Multitargeted	DMM	Phase II	

ANP - antineoplaston, BCR-ABL - BCR-ABL tyrosine kinase, DMM - DNA methylation modifying agent, EGFR - epidermal growth factor receptor, m-TOR - mammalian target of rapamycin, PKC-β2 - protein kinase C-β2, RAS - *RAS* oncogene, TKI - tyrosine-kinase inhibitors, VEGF - vascular endothelial growth factor.

The agents developed by our team, antineoplastons (ANP) are multitargeted therapeutics [20]. Four of these agents A10I (Atengenal), AS2-1I (Astugenal), A10 (Cengenal) and AS2-1 (Fengenal) are the subject of extensive clinical trials which are described in this chapter.

Pharmacological Targets for Currently Used Agents

Formation of brain tumor originates from dysfunction of many different regulatory pathways which consists of increased function of oncogenes and loss of the activity of tumor suppressor genes. Genetic and epigenetic mechanisms produce amplification, or over-expression of growth factors and their receptors, including epidermal growth factor (EGF), platelet-derived growth factor (PDGF), vascular endothelial growth factor (VEGF), and transforming growth factor β1 (TGFBI). Beyond the membrane receptors, a number of oncogenes and tumor suppressor genes are involved in intracellular signal transduction and protection of neoplastic cells from apoptosis. The most important genes for the design of targeted therapy are oncogenes *RAS, AKT, mTOR, MYCC* and *MDM2*, and tumor suppressors *TP53, NF1,* $p21^{Clp1WAF1}$ *(p21), PTEN,* and *INI1*. Finally, exploring differences in cellular and nuclear transport between normal and neoplastic cell may indicate additional targets for new agents.

Inhibition of Growth Factor Signaling

Interruption of signal transduction originating from activation of EGFR, PDGF receptor (PDGFR), VEGF receptor (VEGFR) and TGFBI receptor (TGFBR1) served as the basis for the design of a number of target-oriented agents.

EGFR

EGFR/ERBB1 is a member of a subclass 1 family of the receptor tyrosine kinase (RTK), which comprises of three additional members: ERBB2, ERBB3 and ERBB4 [21]. The receptors consist of three major parts: an extracellular region which binds ligands, a membrane-spanning region and RTK domain in the cytoplasm. The ligands which bind EGFR include EGF, transforming growth factor-α (TGFA), amphiregulin, betacellulin, epiregulin, and heparin-binding EGF. After ligand binding, EGFR forms homo- and heterodimers which leads to activation of RTK, and triggers intracellular signaling.

In gliomas, EGFR is activated by mutation, amplification, and paracrine or autocrine biosynthesis of EGF and other ligands [22]. The most common change of EGFR is amplification which occurs in approximately 50% of primary GBM [23]. Such alteration is less common in low grade glioma. EGFR amplification is frequently associated with mutation in the extracellular domain, known as EGFRvIII variant [24]. This mutation which consists of a 5' deletion of codons 6-273, and allows activation without ligand binding, is found in 67% of EGFR positive tumors [25]. As much as 1/3 of GBM have multiple secondary changes which are associated with amplification and mutation of the *EGFR* [22]. Abnormalities of

EGFR increase tumor invasiveness through up-regulation of matrix metalloproteinases (MMPs) and decrease of apoptosis through activation of BCL-X_L [26, 27].

A group of agents which target EGFR is subject of phase II trials in brain tumors. Small molecules, gefitinib and erlotinib, are competitive specific and reversible inhibitors of the ATP binding to the catalytic site of RTK of the intracellular domain of EGFR. Gefinitib was initially approved in Japan in 2002 and in the U.S. in May 2003 for the treatment of advanced non-small cell lung cancer after failure of other therapies [28]. Gefinitib inhibits receptor autophosphorylation and interrupts intracellular signal transduction. In animal tests using athymic mice with overexpression of EGFR in brain tumors, gefitinib substantially reduced EGFR phosphorylation and increased median survival by approximately 90% [29]. Its action, however, is limited only to cells with EGFR amplification, without EGFRvIII mutation [30]. Erlotinib shares similar mechanisms of action with gefinitib. It has been approved in the U.S. in November 2004 for the treatment of advanced non-small cell lung cancer after failure of at least one prior chemotherapy regimen, and contributed to increase in survival in phase III trials [31]. Erlotinib underwent only limited preclinical testing in brain tumors. The results of phase II trials of gefitinib and erlotinib in high grade gliomas are described in this chapter.

PDGFR

PDGFR and its ligand PDGF play an important part in pathogenesis of gliomas. The PDGFR is a protein tyrosine kinase receptor. Chemically, it is a glycoprotein and contains extracellular, transmembrane and intracellular domains [32]. The external domain binds PDGF ligand which leads to dimerization and autophosphorylation of tyrosine residues in intracellular domains. This creates the sites for the attachment of factors instrumental in signal transduction through important pathways, including RAS, AKT and STAT [33]. PDGFR exists in two forms, α and β, and PDGF in four forms: A, B, C and D. Both PDGFR and PDGF form dimers of various chains (homo- and heterodimers) [22, 32, 34]. PDGFR and PDGF play an important function in the development of the central nervous system, and they are necessary for normal gliogenesis and myelination [35]. Aberrant upregulation of the genes seems to be the main factor which increases expression of PDGFR and PDGF. Another important factor is autocrine stimulation which occurs early in formation of brain tumors and leads to PDGFR expression in most cases [32, 34, 36, 37]. PDGF-A and B are expressed in all gliomas. There is reduced expression of PDGF-A in low grade gliomas, but it is markedly increased in GBM. To the contrary, there is marked expression of PDGFR-α in low and high grade gliomas. PDGFR β is expressed at low levels in all grades.

Imatinib mesylate is the first RTK inhibitor which was successfully introduced for the treatment of chronic myelogenous leukemia and gastrointestinal stromal tumors (GISTs). By interfering with binding of ATP to RTK, imatinib interrupts signal transduction mediated by PDGFR, BCR-ABL, and c-kit [38]. Cell culture and animal tests confirmed activity of imatinib against GBM [39]. The rationale for the use of imatinib in the treatment of brain tumors is based on blocking the activity of not only mutant BCR-ABL and c-kit, but also PDGFR-α kinase [40]. The results of phase II trials are described in this chapter.

VEGFR

The growth of solid tumor is dependent on formation of new blood vessels [41]. VEGF which was isolated as a factor which stimulates endothelial cell division plays a pivotal role in angiogenesis of brain tumors [42]. VEGF family consists of ABCDF and E members, and VEGF-A has at least four isoforms [43]. The members of VEGF family are glycoproteins which form homodimers and bind three different receptors: fms-like tyrosine kinase (FLT1/VEGFR1), kinase insert domain-containing receptor (KDR/VEGFR2), and fetal liver kinase (murine KDR/FLK1) [42, 43]. The receptors are expressed on endothelial and some neoplastic cells. Other stimulators of angiogenesis include fibroblast growth factor (FGF), PDGF and hypoxia-inducible factor 1 (HIF-1). HIF-1 is αβ heterodimer. The HIF-1α transcription factor is stabilized in the absence of oxygen, but HIF-1β occurs at uniform levels in the nucleus. In hypoxic conditions, HIF-1α accumulates in the nucleus, forms heterodimers with a β subunit, and initiates transcription of genes instrumental in angiogenesis and metastasis; among them VEGF [44].

Bevacizumab is a humanized monoclonal antibody against VEGF, which was approved by the U.S. FDA in February 2004 as the first-line treatment of metastatic colorectal cancer, in combination with 5-fluorouracil [45]. Initially, it has been contraindicated in the treatment of brain tumors due to the possibility of intracerebral hemorrhage. Recently conducted phase II trial in high grade glioma is described in this chapter.

TGFBRI

The transforming growth factor β, may have both positive and negative effect on brain tumor progression. It inhibits early stages of neoplastic processes through apoptosis and arrest of G1-S cell cycle transition, but promotes the late stages through angiogenesis and metastasis [46]. TGFB is a polypeptide which exists in three versions: TGF- β1, β2 and β3. TGFB belongs to a super family of more than 30 ligands which are produced by many different kinds of cells, and also include activins, inhibins and bone morphogenic proteins [47]. They are polypeptides which have a common cluster of conserved cysteine residues connected by intramolecular disulfide bonds. TGFB is a product of the gene located on chromosome 19q, and is proteolytically cleaved to 25 kd size. TGFB is bound by TGFB-binding protein and is released by thrombospondin-1, or plasmin [22]. TGFB binds to receptor complex consisting of type I and II (TGFBRI and TGFBRII). The receptors which are serine-threonine kinases are activated by TGFB binding to TGFBRII, which phosphorylates TGFBRI in a glycine-serine-rich region (GS box) [48]. Activated TGFBRI promotes signal transmission through a number of different signaling pathways [46]. They can be grossly divided into Smad and non-Smad pathways. Currently, there are over 10 different Smad proteins which are homologs of the *Sma* and *Mad* genes of *Drosophila melanogaster* and *Caenorhabditis elegans*. The complex consisting of TGFB, TGFBRI and TGFBRII binds to the complex of Smad2, Smad3 and Smad-anchor for receptor activation (SARA) and phosphorylates Smad2 and Smad3. The phosphorylation releases Smad2/3 from a cytoplasmic protein and allows binding to Smad4 and migration into the nucleus [48]. Inside the nucleus, Smad2-4 complex regulates the transcription of numerous genes [46]. Among others it induces *INK4b* (*p15)* and *p21*, and represses *MYCC* and *cyclin-A*. The transmission in TGFB pathway is affected not only by Smad proteins, but also through other pathways, including phosphoinositide 3-kinase (PI3K)/AKT and mitogen-activated protein kinase p38 (p38 MAPK) [49]. Smads play an important part in TGFBs growth inhibition and apoptosis, but p38 and PI3K/AKT regulate transcription and motility [50]. The abnormalities in TGFB/Smad signaling pathway promote neoplastic growth and can occur through mutations of *TGFBRI, TGFBRII, SMAD2 and SMAD4*, which leads to the loss of expression of TGFB1 receptors and Smads. The increased activity of TGFB1 makes neoplastic cells more aggressive, and increases angiogenesis. The role played by TGFB in pathogenesis of gliomas is not completely understood [51]. TGFB is released by high grade glioma cells which also express the receptors [52]. GBM cells are expressing TGFBRI/II and TGFB2 at a higher level than low grade gliomas [53]. On the other hand, Smad2-4 are expressed at a lower level in some high grade glioma [54]. TGFB also down-regulates expression of PTEN [55].

Pre-clinical tests confirm the validity of targeted therapy directed against TGFBI [51, 56]. PG, which is the main ingredient of A10I, decreases expression of TGFB1, and shows activity against brain tumors in phase II studies as described later in this chapter [57, 58]. (Figure 2)

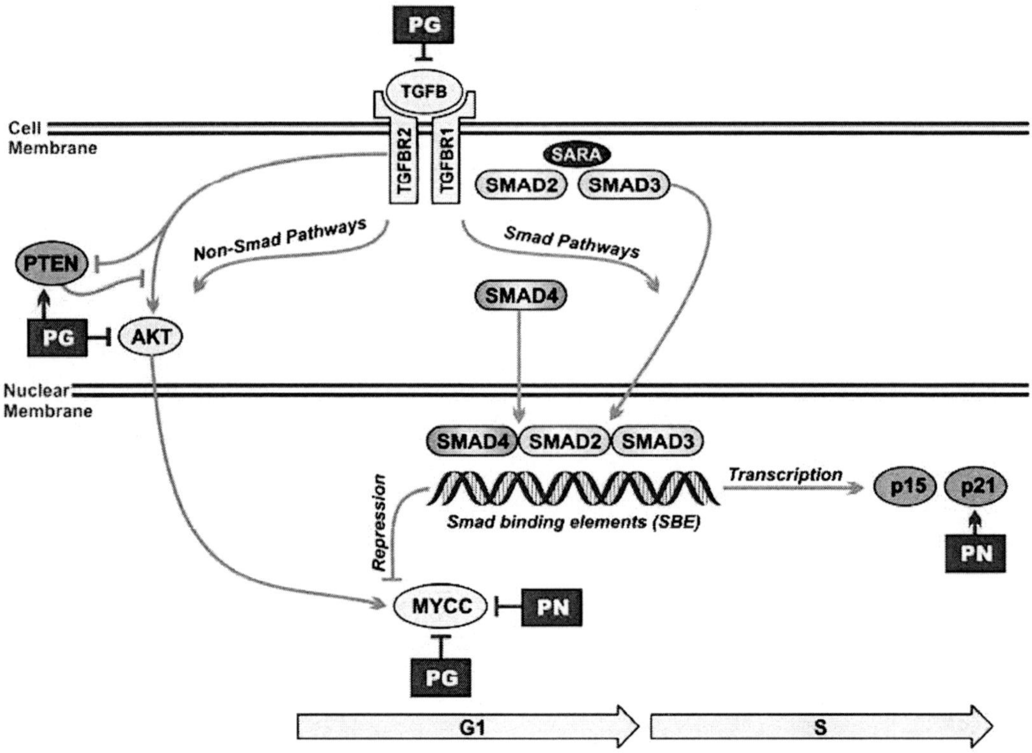

Figure 2. Pharmaceutical agents targeting transforming growth factor β signaling. TGFB, TGFBR1, TGFBR2 - transforming growth factor β, and its receptors, SMAD2, 3, 4 – Smad proteins, SARA – Smad – anchor for receptor activation, PTEN, p15, p21 - tumor suppressor gene proteins, AKT, MYCC – oncogene proteins, PG – phenylacetylglutaminate sodium, ingredient of ANP A10I, PN – phenylacetate sodium, main ingredient of ANP AS2-1I.

Inhibition of Signal Transduction Pathway Intermediates

The most important signaling pathways in the treatment of brain tumors are RAS and PI3K/AKT. These pathways can transmit signals from any of the ligand-receptor systems described before.

RAS

RAS proteins and MAPK form one of the most important signaling systems for cell proliferation. It receives signals from growth factors receptors and transmits them to cell nucleus [59]. The main position in the pathway is occupied by RAS protein which is guanosine triphosphatase (GTPase) RAS. In mammals, there are four RAS proteins HRAS, NRAS and KRAS 4A and KRAS4B, which are the products of 3 genes [60]. *KRAS* gene is most frequently mutated (approximately 80-85% of total *RAS* mutation). *NRAS* and *HRAS* are mutated in lesser percentage of cases (correspondingly, 15% and 1%) [61]. The proteins which are products of oncogenes located on chromosomes 11p, 12p and 1p respectively encode very similar molecules but with different carboxyl termini. RAS proteins require modification through farnesylation, proteolytic cleavage, carboxymethylation and palmitoylation. NRAS and KRAS4A are acylated with one palmitoyl residue, HRAS with two and KRAS4B contains C-terminal polybasic amino acids instead of palmitoyl moiety [62]. The most important step in activation of RAS is farnesylation facilitated by farnesyltransferase (FTase), which attaches 15 carbon isoprenoid fragment. RAS functions at the plasma membrane and in Golgi complex [63]. Palmitoylated proteins are present in the Golgi and at the membrane; whereas, KRAS4B is attached only to the membrane. In this respect, there are two signaling platforms, membrane and the Golgi, but it is not known at present how these pathways are segregated [64]. Since RAS is involved in fundamentally different processes, proliferation and differentiation, its distribution to two cellular compartments may explain diverse aspects of the activity. The advantage of the Golgi location is the proximity of the nucleus which is at the receiving end of the signal [62]. At the membrane, RAS GDP is rapidly converted to RAS GTP as the result of binding ligands to growth factor receptors described earlier in this chapter. Adapter protein GRB2 binds SH2 domains of autophosphorylated receptor and conduct the signal to RAS guanine-nucleotide exchange factors (GEFs). After binding SH2 domains of GRB2, GEF activates RAS through the exchange of GDP to GTP. RAS GTP conducts signals to numerous effectors which are responsible for the variety of biological activities: transcription (RAF/MEK/ERK), cell cycle progression (PI3K/AKT) translation (PI3K/PDK1) apoptosis (RASSF-1), cell-cell junctions (AF6), endocytosis (RIN1), membrane (RAL) and nuclear transport (PLCε) [59]. In addition to various GEFs (the best known are SOS1/2), there are numerous naturally occurring inhibitors of RAS activation. RTK is inhibited by SPROUTY and ACK, which bind GRB2, and a number of GTPase-activaging proteins (GAPs). Among them is neurofibromin, the product of neurofibromatosis 1 gene (*NF1*). In this respect, inactivation of *NF1* activates RAS [65].

RAS gene is frequently mutated in human cancers (in approximately 30% of all cancers). Mutated *RAS* is losing sensitivity to hydrolysis catalyzed by GAP, which results in increased signal transmission. The mutations are rare in gliomas, but increased activity of RASGTP was found in GBM, and high grade astrocytomas [22, 66, 67]. It is generally accepted that the activation of RAS signaling in brain tumors is due to increased activity of receptors RTKs.

Agents which inhibit farnesylation of RAS have shown efficacy and low toxicity in pre-clinical and clinical studies [68]. The beneficial results, however, were limited to hematological malignancies [69]. Such agents fell short of expectations in the treatment of solid tumors [70]. The inhibitor of farnesyltransferase, lonafarnib has been used in phase II studies of GBM, and the results are described in this chapter. One of the reasons for failure of these agents is "alternative prenylation" which permits modification of KRAS by geranylgeranyltransferase-1 (GGTase-1) [71, 72]. The alternative inhibition of farnesylation of RAS can be obtained through depletion of isoprenoids in cells [70]. This can be accomplished by inhibition of 5-pyrophosphomevalonate decarboxylase by PN (main ingredient of ANP AS2-1I) [73]. Interruption of signal transduction downstream of RAS protein creates interesting targets for anticancer agents. Based on the studies in breast cancer cell line, PG and isoPG (ingredients of A10I) inhibit phosphorylation of ERK [74]. The results of phase II trials with ANP are described in this chapter. (Figure 3)

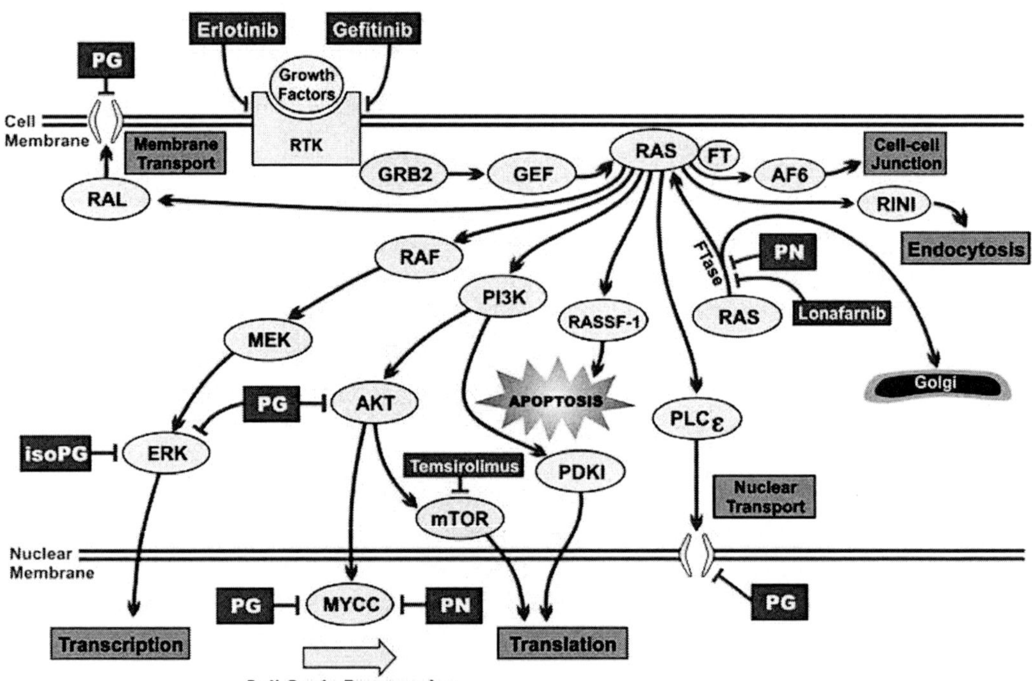

Figure 3. Pharmaceutical agents targeting RAS signaling pathway. RTK – receptor tyrosine kinase, GRB2 – adapter protein, GEF - guanine – nucleotide exchange factor, RAS – *RAS* oncogene protein, RASFT – farnesylated *RAS* protein, AF6, RIN1, RAL, RAF, RASSF-1, PLCε, MEK, ERK – RAS effectors, PI3K, AKT, mTOR, MYCC – oncogene proteins, PG – phenylacetylglutaminate sodium, ingredient of ANP A10I, isoPG – phenylacetyisoglutaminate sodium – ingredient of ANP A10I, PN – phenylacetate sodium, main ingredient of ANP AS2-1I.

PI3K/AKT

PI3K/AKT pathway is of primary importance in pathogenesis of brain tumors [66]. The signal orginates from activation of PI3K which can be accomplished by numerous growth factor receptors and RAS pathway. The most important include insulin-like growth factor 1 receptor (IGF-1R), EGFR, PDGFR and VEGFR [75]. Second messengers generated by PI3K, phosphatidylinositols (PtdIns): PtdIns (4,5) P_2 (PIP_2) and PtdIns (3,4,5) P_3 (PIP_3) recruit AKT (which is serine-threonine kinase)to the cell membrane. AKT family includes three members: AKT1, AKT2 and AKT3, which are phosphorylated by 3-phosphoinositide-dependent protein kinase – 1 (PDK1) and PDK2. PIP_3 is inactivated through conversion to PIP_2 by phosphatase and tensine homolog (PTEN). This mechanism resembles inactivation of RASGTP by GAPs. AKT activates and inhibits numerous targets. Through activation of mTOR it promotes cell cycle progression, initiation of translation and survival. Inhibition of BAD and FOXO factors, and activation of NFκB by AKT blocks apoptosis. This is also accomplished through increased activity of MDM2 which inhibits p53 [76]. High grade gliomas show increased activity of PI3K/AKT pathway but amplification of AKT has not yet been described in human astrocytomas [77, 78]. The main mechanism is inactivation of PTEN, which is deleted in the majority of high grade gliomas, and increased activity of EGFR, PDGFR and RAS signaling [22, 78]. Increased activity of AKT is mediated in substantial degree by mTOR, especially when there is a loss of PTEN [79]. The impact of mTOR pathway is substantial in maintaining the transformed phenotype of cancer cells, but mTOR mutations, or overexpression, have not yet been reported in human cancers [76]. mTOR inhibitor temsirolimus has been used in phase II trials of recurrent GBM. PG, which is the main ingredient of ANP A10I, decreases expression of AKT2 and activates PTEN (through inhibition of TGFB1) [57, 58]. The results of phase II studies of temsirolimus and ANP are described in this chapter. (Figure 4)

Inhibition of G1-S Transition

Progression of neoplastic process requires continuous cell divisions which occur in mitosis (M) phase of cell cycle. Before mitosis occurs, the cell must replicate its DNA in synthesis (S) phase. Two additional phases separate S and M. In G1 phase between the end of mitosis and beginning of DNA synthesis, the decision is made within the cell to replicate its DNA or rest. In G2 phase (between S and M phases) the cell activates the mechanisms which prevent mitosis in case of DNA damage and delay cell division until the damage is repaired. At G1-S checkpoint, the cell is under influence of numerous signaling pathways. Among these pathways RAS and PI3K/AKT are the most important. Transition from G1 to S and initiation of DNA synthesis would not occur unless there is activation of cyclin-dependent kinases 2 and 4 (CDK2/4). In order to accomplish their tasks, CDKs form active catalytic complexes with cyclins; CDK2 with cyclins E1, E2 and A, and CDK4 and, CDK6 with cyclins of D type. At the beginning of G1, *MYCC* oncogene through MYC-MAX dimers activates genes *CDK4* and *CCND2*, which express CDK4 and cyclin D2 [80, 81]. *MYC*

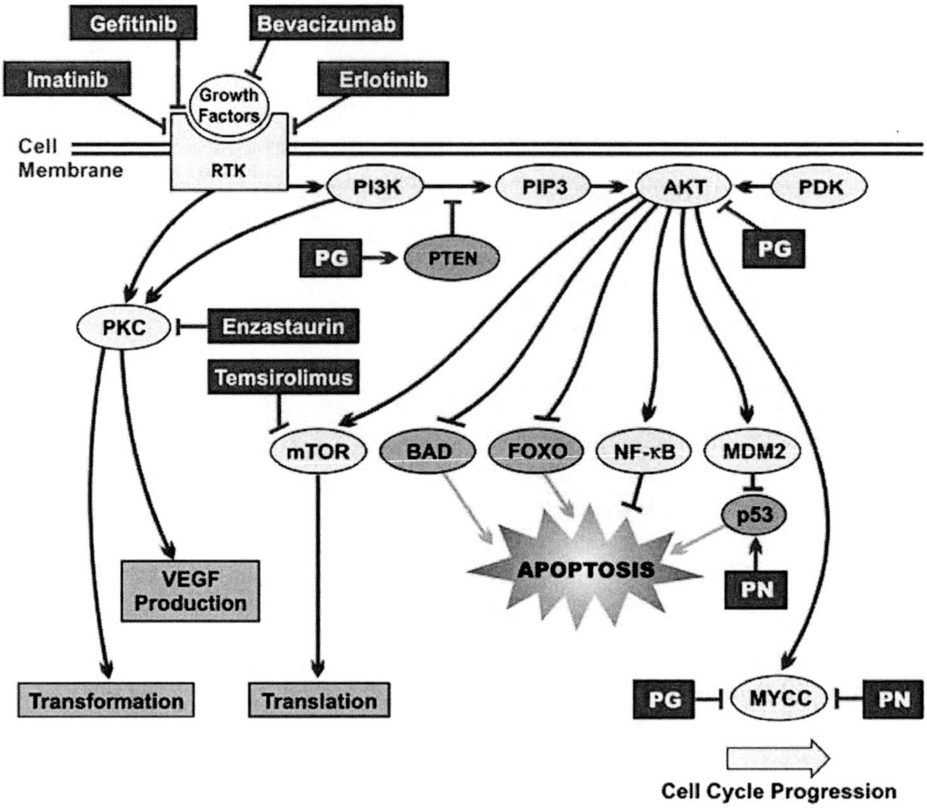

Figure 4. Pharmaceutical agents targeting PI3K/AKT signaling pathway. RTK- receptor tyrosine kinase, PI3K - phosphoinositide 3-kinase, PIP3 -phosphatidylinositol 3,4,5, PDK – phosphoinositide-dependent protein kinase, AKT – serine-threonine kinase, product of AKT oncogene, mTOR-mammalian target of rapamycin, BAD-apoptosis inducing protein, FOXO, NF-κB, MDM2, MYCC - oncogene proteins, p53 – p53 protein, PG – phenylacetylglutaminate sodium, ingredient of ANP A10I, PN – phenylacetate sodium, main ingredient of ANP AS2-1I, VEGF – vascular endothelial growth factor, PKC – protein kinase C-β2.

family of oncogenes (*MYCC, MYCL* and *MYCN)* play an extremely important part in regulation of G1-S transition [82, 83]. These oncogenes are over-expressed in over 50% of all malignancies, usually through epigenetic mechanisms and interact directly and indirectly with close to a thousand targets. MYC proteins are stabilized and activated by phosphorylation of serine 62 (Ser 62). Degradation (ubiquitination) of MYC is facilitated by phosphorylation of threonine 58 (Thr58) [84]. These processes are regulated by RAS and AKT signaling. In RAS pathway, the cascade of events (RAF1/extracellular signal-regulated kinase-ERK) affects phosphorylation (activation) of MYC at Ser 62 [85]. AKT prevents MYC degradation through inhibition of glycogen synthase3- β (GSK3-β), and phosphorylation of Thr58 [83]. Complex cyclin D/CDK4 binds and commit to ubiquitination an inhibitor of CDK2-KIP1 (p27) [86]. KIP1 serves also as an inhibitor of G1-S transition, and its inactivation is promoted by two genes, *CUL-1* and *CKS*, targeted by MYC [87]. In this respect, inhibition of MYC prevents formation of cyclin D2/CDK4 complex and inactivation of KIP1. Such inhibition can be accomplished through interruption of RAS and AKT signaling and MAD family proteins [81]. Neutralization of KIP1 activity eliminates inhibition of cyclin E/CDK2 complex. Elevated concentrations of cyclin E are necessary for entering S phase [88]. The expression of cyclin E is regulated by E2F factors [89]. At the beginning of G1 these factors are sequestrated by the retinoblastoma protein (Rb), and its related proteins p107 and p130. E2F1, E2F2 and E2F3 are inactivated, whereas, E2F4 and E2F5 become repressors [89]. Rb is inactivated through phosphorylation by complexes cyclin D/CDK4 and cyclin D/CDK6 [90]. Phosphorylation releases E2F from Rb binding and allows its function as a transcription factor for cyclin E, DNA polymerase α and other proteins necessary for DNA replication. Additional inhibitors of cyclin/CDK complexes are INK4A (p16), p15 and p21. p15 and p21 inhibit cyclin E/CDK2 and arrest cell cycle progression [91]. MYC-MAX together with MYC-interacting zinc finger protein 1 (MIZ1) blocks activation of *CDKN1A* and *CDKN2B* which are genes encoding p21 and p15 correspondingly. Cyclin D1/CDK4 is inhibited by p16 which is activated by INI1 tumor suppressor gene protein. On the other hand, AKT2 phosphorylation of GSK3-β prevents inactivation of cyclin D (phosphorylation of cyclin D by GSK3- β causes its destabilization) [92].

ANP affects multiple targets at G1-S transition. The mechanisms involving RAS and AKT signaling pathways were described previously [20, 57, 58, 73]. In addition, PN, PG and isoPG activate p21and PG increases expression of MAD through MADS box transcription enhancer factor (MEFD2D) [57, 58, 74, 81, 93]. PG and isoPG increase the expression of p16 [74]. (Figure 5)

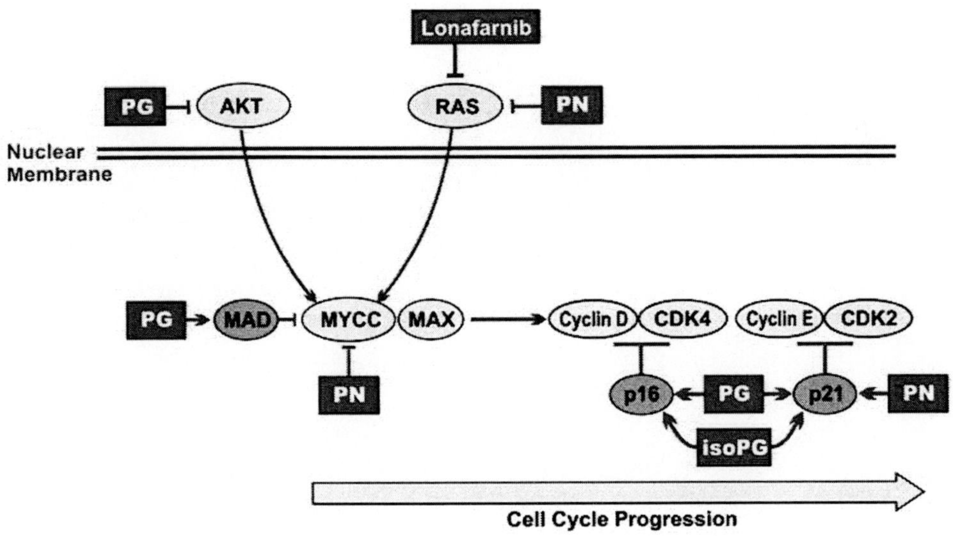

Figure 5. Pharmaceutical agents targeting G1-S transition. AKT, RAS, MYCC, MAX – oncogene proteins, CDK2 – cyclin-dependent kinase 2, MAD, p16, p21 – tumor suppressor gene proteins, PG – phenylacetylglutaminate sodium, ingredient of ANP A10I, isoPG - phenylacetyisoglutaminate sodium, ingredient of ANP A10I, PN – phenylacetate sodium, main ingredient of ANP AS2-1I.

Induction of Apoptosis

Induction of neoplastic cell death is the final goal of any targeted therapy, but some regimens used in treatment of brain tumors, explore also direct apoptotic mechanisms. Apoptosis is a highly complex process and it is the subject of numerous excellent reviews [82, 94-98]. It proceeds through two main pathways. Extrinsic pathway leads through CD95 receptor, tumor necrosis factor (TNF) and TNF-related apoptosis-inducing ligand (TRAIL) [99-101]. The main event in the second (intrinsic) pathway is the release of cytochrome c from mitochondria [102]. The extrinsic and intrinsic pathways are united in the common cascade of activation of proteolytic enzymes, caspases, which together with cytochrome c and apoptotic protease-activating factor 1 (APAF1) form apoptosome (wheel of death) and degrade proteins. Proteins of BCL-2 family play an important part in regulation of apoptosis. Anti-apoptotic proteins, BCL-2 and BCL-X_L inhibit pro-apoptotic BAX. Proteins BAX and BAD promote mitochondrial-outer-membrane permeabilization (MOMP) and release of cytochrome c. BAD is inhibited by RAS and AKT, and BAX is activated by p53 [82]. p53 protein plays a central role in this process, and its loss leads to inhibition of apoptosis [94, 103, 104]. Through transactivation of p21, p53 protein causes arrest of the cell cycle at G1-S checkpoint, and is also instrumental in transcription of many apoptosis-associated genes including *BAX* [105-107].

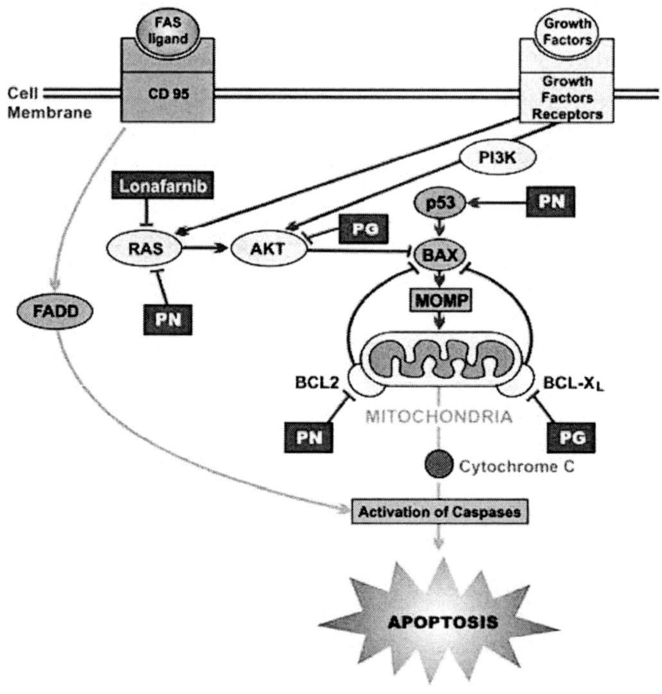

Figure 6. Induction of apoptosis by targeted pharmaceuticals. CD95 – CD95 receptor, PI3K, AKT, RAS – oncogene proteins, p53 – p53 protein, BAX – pro-apoptotic protein, FADD – intracellular adapter protein (FAS-associated death domain), MOMP – mitochondrial-outer-membrane permeabilization, BCL2, BCL-$_{XL}$ – anti-apoptotic proteins, PG - phenylacetylglutaminate sodium, ingredient of ANP A10I, PN - phenylacetate sodium, ingredient of ANP AS2-1I.

ANP are among agents used in phase II studies of brain tumors, which directly target apoptotic machinery. PN increases expression of p53 and p21, and inhibits BCL-2 [108-110]. PG inhibits BCL-X_L [57, 58]. Indirectly, PN and PG promote apoptosis of neoplastic cells through interruption of signal transmission in RAS and AKT pathways [20, 57, 58, 73]. (Figure 6)

Inhibition of Membrane Transport

Cellular Membrane Transport

Active cancer growth requires effective transport of molecules through the cell membrane and also continuous shuttling of signaling proteins between nucleus and cytoplasm. Differences in membrane transport may create targets for anti-cancer drugs and they are utilized in ANP therapy of brain tumors. PG inhibits the uptake of growth-critical amino acids, such as L-glutamine and L-leucine in glioma cells [20, 57]. PG enters cells via the stereo-specific amino acid transporters for L-glutamine, decreases intracellular concentrations of L-glutamine and L-leucine, which contributes to anti-neoplastic activity.

Nuclear Transport

Important signaling molecules move back and forth between the cytoplasm and nucleus. The nuclear localization of the products of important tumor suppressor genes *TP53* and *INI1* is necessary for their function. The mutation of INI1 gene plays a crucial part in development of atypical teratoid/rhabdoid tumor (AT/RT), and some cases of GBM [111, 112]. INI1 represses transcription of cyclin D1 and induces p16, blocking G1-S cell-cycle transition. Mutation of the *INI1* gene at 22q11 effects nuclear export signal and causes INI protein to migrate to the cytoplasm where it is not active [113]. INI1 transport from the nucleus to the cytoplasm also depends on RanGTP/RanGDP gradient, and Ran binding protein 1 (RanBP1), which causes increased concentration of RanGDP in the cytoplasm. PG decreases expression of RanBP1 and prevents escape of INI1 from the nucleus [57, 58, 114].

Modification of Epigenetic Changes

Aberrant methylation of promoters of tumor suppressors and decreased global methylation are the most common epigenetic changes occurring in primary brain tumors [12, 115-119]. Increased methylation of promoters causes silencing of numerous genes, including p15 and p16. It is important to note that silencing of p16 occurs in approximately 25% of gliomas and of the tissue inhibitor of metalloproteinase-3 (TIMP-3) in up to 80% [118, 119]. Global hypomethylation is very common and was found in both low and high grade tumors. It is causing genomic instability, amplification of oncogenes, multi-drug resistance, and is more pronounced in high grade tumors [119-121]. Mutation of *INI1*, which is part of SWI/SNF complex contributes to hypomethylation. Methylation is associated with chromatin remodeling and histone modification [122, 123]. Acetylation of lysine in histone tails loosens compact chromatin structures and allows gene expression. The reverse process –

deacetylation catalyzed by histone deacetylase (HDAC) blocks gene expression. Pharmacological agents which modify abberant DNA methylation and histone acetylation create attractive possibilities for the treatment of brain tumors. Unfortunately, most of currently used agents lack specificity. The first drug in this group, azacitidine, an inhibitor of DNA methylation, was approved by U.S. F.D.A. for the treatment of myelodysplastic syndromes in May, 2004 [124].

ANP normalizes aberrant DNA methylation. PG affects global hypomethylation and PN decreases methylation of the promoters of tumor suppressor genes and inhibits HDAC [2, 58, 115].

Phase II Clinical Studies of Targeted Therapy in Brain Tumors

Treatment of High Grade Glioma

High grade gliomas (HGGs) represent approximately 60% of primary brain tumors and include GBM, AA, anaplastic oligodendroglioma and anaplastic oligoastrocytoma. GBM is clinically most important and affects approximately 12,500 patients in the U.S. [125]. With traditional treatment, median survival is 9-10 months with most patients dying within 2 years [126]. Standard treatment for newly diagnosed GBM consists of surgical resection followed by radiation therapy. Adjuvant chemotherapy with nitrosourea did not produce a survival benefit according to randomized phase III trial of 674 patients [127]. The prognosis is even poorer for recurrent high grade glioma with median survival of approximately 7 months for chemotherapy [128]. Introduction of TMZ raised hopes for more successful treatment [129, 130]. Phase II study of TMZ versus procarbazine in patients with GBM at first relapse confirmed improved overall survival (OS), progression-free survival (PFS), as well as percentage of objective response in patients treated with TMZ [131]. Phase III trial involving 573 patients with newly diagnosed GBM compared overall survival of patients treated with radiation therapy alone versus radiotherapy plus concomitant and adjuvant TMZ[10]. The addition of TMZ to radiotherapy for newly diagnosed GBM produced statistically better survival with low toxicity. The results of recent trials are summarized in Table 2.

Imatinib successfully introduced for the treatment of chronic myeloid leukemia has been tested in a number of different phase II studies in recurrent GBM and AA as a single agent or in addition to hydroxyurea [132-135] . In studies with imatanib as a single agent, there was no significant benefit measured as PFS and objective response. Combination treatment with hydroxyurea provided better results with 3% of complete response (CR), 13% of partial response (PR), 37% of stable disease (SD) and 32% of PFS at 6 months [134]. Gefitinib was tested in recurrent GBM with no confirmed objective responses and PFS at 6 months from 12 to 14% [136, 137]. Additional 2 separate phase II studies with erlotinib in recurrent GBM produced better results. Vogelbaum, et al. reported 21% PR in 24 patients and Cloughesy et al., 2% of CR and 6% of PR in 48 patients [138, 139]. Bevacizumab in combination with irinotecan was administered to 21 patients with relapsed high grade glioma in recently reported phase II study [140]. The results consisting of 5% CR and 38% PR were encouraging. Farnesyltransferase inhibitor, lonafarnib, was administered in combination with TMZ to 23 patients with recurrent GBM, and contributed to 13% of PR and 44% of SD. PFS at 6 months was 13% which was higher in procarbazine but lower than TMZ study [141]. mTor inhibitor, temsirolimus and PKC-β2 inhibitor, enzastaurin did not produce significant responses in phase II studies in recurrent GBM and HGG [142, 143]

ANP therapy was studied in phase II trials of 22 patients with relapsed GBM, and contributed to 9% of CR and PR, 54.5% of SD and PFS at 6 months of 50% [144]. The analysis of the results of treatment of 173 evaluable patients with recurrent and progressed GBM in phase II trials with ANP have shown significant percentage of response rates and long-term survival (LTS) [145]. Seventy-nine of these patients were treated in the study protocols and an additional 94 patients were treated under special exception (SE) due to low Karnofsky Performance Status (KPS) below 60. 98% of patients failed prior surgery, radiation therapy and/or chemotherapy [145]. LTS was defined as survival more than 3 years after the initial diagnosis of GBM. For patients in the study group (SP), the LTS was 15.5% and in SE group was 7.1%. The maximum survival in SP was more than 13 years and in SE was more than 10 years. The results of targeted therapy in GBM and HGG, including additional data on ANP, are summarized in Table 3.

Treatment of Brain Stem Glioma

Brain stem gliomas (BSGs) are among the most difficult to treat brain tumors. They are relatively uncommon and constitute less than 10% of all primary tumors of the central nervous system [146, 147]. Approximately 80% of these tumors occur in children and 20% in adult patients. Based on MRI appearance they are usually classified in four different types: focal, dorsal exophytic, cervicomedullary and diffuse intrinsic (DBSG) [148]. DBSGs, which occur in 85% of cases, are the most difficult to treat. This is, however, not a homogenous group. These tumors have different histopathology and different clinical course, depending on the age of the patient. In infants, DBSG is more aggressive, but on the other hand it has as slower clinical course in patients between the ages of 22 to 39, and when it is associated with neurofibromatosis type I [147]. Patients over the age of 40 have worse prognosis and higher percentage of GBM (over 30%). Based on autopsy results, the majority of patients have AA. There is a lower incidence of a low-grade astrocytoma and GBM. Close to 50% of young adults less than 40 years of age have low-grade glioma [147]. It should be noted that only approximately 25% of BSG patients have a biopsy and that histopathology diagnosis is not accurate due to difficulty in securing sufficient size of sample in a strategic area of brain. It is also possible that a specimen taken from one area of the tumor does not represent histopathology of the area which was not biopsied. It is a general consensus of neuro-oncologists that all DBSG should be treated as high-grade gliomas. On the other hand, the remaining three types of BSG usually have histopathological diagnosis and are treated the same way as tumors in other parts of the brain. The aggressive behaviour of DBSG is manifested also by dissemination through cerebrospinal fluid in approximately 20% of cases. The data on genetic abnormalities in DBSG are quite limited, but they indicate that in more than 30% of these patients, EGFR protein is detected and half of these patients have *TP53* mutated [149]. *EGFR* gene is amplified only in some patients, and in half of the cases there is loss of *PTEN* [150, 151].

DBSG are non-resectable. Radiation therapy is the main treatment for newly diagnosed tumors [152]. A number of studies confirmed that standard radiation therapy is preferable over hyperfractionation and combination with chemotherapy [152, 153]. The prognosis is poor with approximately 7% survival at 2 years and no survival over 5 years in most of the studies [147, 152, 153]. Numerous chemotherapy regimens including TMZ given before, concomitant and after radiation therapy and high-dose treatment with autologous bone marrow transplantation did not improve the results and contributed to toxicity [154-162]. The prognosis is especially poor for recurrent DBSG with no standard chemotherapy available, including TMZ [11]. Patients with recurrent DBSG usually do not survive longer than 6 months, despite the treatment given.

Therapy, which affects single targets, was not yet studied in DBSG, but multitargeted therapy with ANP shows promising results [163-167]. Phase II studies of ANP are nearing completion. The results, which were recently reported, were based on the total of 65 evaluable patients [165]. The majority of the patients (72%) developed relapsed DBSG after standard therapy and 28% had progressive DBSG without prior treatment. The condition of 35 patients was not satisfactory for the admission to clinical studies (KPS from 40-50), which required SE from the FDA. Two thirds of these patients did not have a biopsy due to the dangerous location of the tumor, but in the remaining group of patients, 3 were diagnosed with GBM, 8 with AA, 5 with astrocytoma, 3 with pilocytic astrocytoma, 1 with oligodendroglioma, 1 with anaplastic mixed glioma and 1 with glioma. The results in comparison with TMZ chemotherapy are shown in Table 4.

Over 40% of the study patients survived over 2 years and 30% over 5 years. CR occurred in 27%, PR in 20%, SD in 23% and progressive disease (PD) in 30% in study patients. Median survival time (MST) for study patients was 20 months.

Another report described the efficacy of ANP in high-grade BSGs [166]. Sixteen patients with inoperable BSG were studied, including 4 with GBM and 12 with AA. In 9 cases, the tumor relapsed and in 1 case persisted after prior treatment and 6 patients did not have radiation therapy or chemotherapy. Thirty-one percent of patients survived over 2 years and 12.5% over 5 years. The maximum survival is over 6 years for recurrent GBM and over 18 years for recurrent AA. Complete and partial responses were obtained in 18.7%, SD in 14% and PD in 37.5%.

Another group of 10 evaluable patients with inoperable BSGs consisted of children less than 4 years' of age [167]. Three of these patients had a biopsy which confirmed 2 cases of AA and one pilocytic astrocytoma. The youngest patient was a 3-month-old infant. Three patients failed prior radiation therapy and chemotherapy. These patients have shown the best survival data; 60% at 2 years, 20% at 5 years and a maximum survival over 7 years. Complete responses were documented in 30%, SD in 40% and PD in 30%.

Table 2. Results of Radiation Therapy in Combination with Chemotherapy for Glioblastoma Multiforme

Author	Study Type		Patients N	Treatment		Efficacy								
				Radiation Therapy	Additional Chemotherapy	OS			MST	PFS 6 M	CR	PR	SD	PD
				Gy		1 yr %	2 yrs %	5 yrs %	M	%	%	%	%	%
Yung et al., 2000 (131)	Phase II	Arm 1	112	None	Temozolomide	25	NA	NA	NA	21	0	5	40	NA
	RGBM	Arm 2	113	None	Procarbazine	15	NA	NA	NA	8	0	5	27	NA
Stupp et al., 2005 (10)	Phase III	Arm 1	286	60	None	50.6	21.2	NA	12.1	36.4	NA	NA	NA	NA
	NGBM	Arm 2	287	60	Temozolomide	61.1	26.5	NA	14.6	53.9	NA	NA	NA	NA

CR - complete response, M - months, MST - median survival time, N - number, NA - not available, - NGBM - newly diagnosed GBM, OS - overall survival, PD - progressive disease, PFS - progression-free survival, PR - partial response, RGBM - recurrent GBM, SD - stable disease

Table 3. Results of Targeted Therapy for Glioblastoma Multiforme and High Grade Glioma

Author	Study Type	Tumor Type	Patients N	Treatment		Efficacy								
				Targeted Therapy	Additional Treatment	OS			MST	PFS 6M	CR	PR	SD	PD
						1 yr %	2 yrs %	5 yrs %	M	%	%	%	%	%
Wen et al. (2004)(132)	Phase II	Total	48	Imatinib	None									
		RGBM	29	Imatinib	None	NA	NA	NA	NA	3	0	3	21	NA
		RAA	19	Imatinib	None	NA	NA	NA	NA	11	0	0	10	NA
van den Bent et al. (2004)(133)	Phase II	RGBM	51	Imatinib	None	NA	NA	NA	NA	NA	0	6	18	NA
Dresemann et al. (2005)(134)	Phase II	RGBM	30	Imatinib	Hydroxyurea	NA	13	NA	NA	32	3	13	37	47
Reardon, et al. (2005)(135)	Phase II	Total	64	Imatinib	Hydroxyurea									
		RGBM	32	Imatinib	Hydroxyurea	NA	NA	NA	NA	26	NA	9	35	NA
		RAA	32	Imatinib	Hydroxyurea	NA	NA	NA	NA	NA	NA	NA	NA	NA
Rich et al. (2004)(136)	Phase II	RGBM*	57	Gefitinib	None	NA	NA	NA	10*	NA	0	0	NA	NA

Table 3. Results of Targeted Therapy for Glioblastoma Multiforme and High Grade Glioma (Continued)

Author	Study Type	Tumor Type	Patients N	Treatment		Efficacy								
				Targeted Therapy	Additional Treatment	OS			MST	PFS 6M	CR	PR	SD	PD
						1 yr %	2 yrs %	5 yrs %	M	%	%	%	%	%
Franceschi et al. (2005)(137)	Phase II	Total	28	Gefitinib	None	NA	NA	NA	NA	14	0	4†	18	NA
		RGBM	16	Gefitinib	None	14	6	NA	NA	12	NA	NA	NA	NA
		RAG	12	Gefitinib	None	NA	NA	NA	NA	NA	NA	NA	NA	NA
Vogelbaum et al. (2004)(138)	Phase II	RGBM	24	Erlotinib	None	NA	NA	NA	NA	NA	0	21	21	42
Cloughesy et al. (2005)(139)	Phase II	RGBM	48	Erlotinib	None	NA	NA	NA	10	17	2	6	37	NA
Stark-Vance (2005)(140)	Phase II	RHG	21	Bevacizumab	Irinotecan	NA	NA	NA	NA	NA	5	38	52	NA
Gilbert et al. (2005)(141)	Phase II	RGBM	23	Lonafarnib	Temozolomide	NA	NA	NA	9	13	0	13	44	NA
Galanis et al. (2005)(142)	Phase II	RGBM	52	Temsirolimus	None	NA	NA	NA	NA	10	0	0	NA‡	NA
Fine et al. (2005)(143)	Phase II	RHG	85	Enzastaurin	None	NA	NA	NA	NA	NA	1§	16§	NA	NA
Weaver et al. (2004)(144)	Phase II	RGBM	22	ANP	None	82	27	5	16.4	50	4.5	4.5	54.5	36.5
Weaver et al. (2005)(145)	Phase II	Total	173	ANP	None	58	19	5	13.5	44	6	8	35	51
Study	Phase II	RGBM	79	ANP	None	65	27	8	15.5	39	9	10	29	52
Special Exception	Phase II	RGBM	94	ANP	None	52	12	3	12.7	48	3	6.5	40.5	50

ANP - antineoplastons A10I and AS2-1I, CR - complete response, M - months, MST - median survival time, N - number, NA - not available, OS - overall survival, PD - progressive disease, PFS - progression-free survival, PR - partial response, RAA - recurrent anaplastic astrocytoma, RAG - recurrent anaplastic glioma, RGBM - recurrent glioblastoma multiforme, RHG - recurrent high grade glioma, SD - stable disease.

* 79% of patients did not have baseline measurable disease

† unconfirmed

‡ 16 patients had evidence of decrease in T2, signal abnormality on MRI,

§ based on 79 evaluable patients

Table 4. Treatment of Recurrent and Progressed Intrinsic Brain Stem Glioma with Temozolomide and ANP

Author	Study Type	Patient N	Treatment	Efficacy						
				OS		MST	CR	PR	SD	PD
				2 yrs %	5 yrs %	M	%	%	%	%
Lashford (11)	Phase II	18	Temozolomide	NA	NA	6.2	0	5.6	16.7	77.8
Burzynski et al. (165)	Phase II		ANP							
Total		65		38.5	21.5	15	20	14	37	29
Study		30		43	30	20	27	20	23	30
Special Exception		35		34	14	13	14	9	48	29

ANP - antineoplastons A10I and AS2-1I, CR - complete response, MST- median time survival, N - number, OS - overall survival, PD - progressive disease, PR - partial response, SD - stable disease

Table 5. Treatment of High-Risk Pediatric Brain Tumor Patients with ANP

Author	Diagnosis	Study Type	Patients N	Efficacy						
				OS		MST	CR	PR	SD	PD
				2 yrs %	5 yrs %	M	% (N)	% (N)	% (N)	% (N)
Burzynski et al. (168)	PNET	Phase II	13	77	46	42	23 (3)	8 (1)	31 (4)	38 (5)
Burzynski et al. (177)	Multicentric Glioma	Phase II	11	100	64	82	36.5 (4)	27 (3)	36.5 (4)	0
Burzynski et al. (114)	AT/RT	Phase II	8	12.5	0	15	25 (2)	12.5 (1)	12.5 (1)	50 (4)

ANP - antineoplastons A10I and AS2-1I, AT/RT - atypical teratoid/rhabdoid tumor, CR - complete response,
PNET - primitive neuroectodermal tumor, M - months, MST - median survival time, N - number,
OS - overall survival, PD - progressive disease, PR - partial response, SD - stable disease.

Treatment of High Risk Pediatric Patients with Primary Brain Tumors

Among pediatric neurooncology patients, there is a substantial incidence of high risk cases. Primitive neuroectodermal tumors (PNETs) are the most common malignancies of the central nervous system in children. They include medulloblastoma, pineoblastoma, supratentorial PNET, and ependymoblastoma [168]. PNET can be successfully treated with surgery, radiation therapy and chemotherapy [169]. Unfortunately, such treatment program is not successful after subtotal resection, dissemination of the disease, age younger than 4 years and certain histopathological and genetic characteristics, including large cell anaplastic variety, and overexpression of MYCC oncogene [170, 171]. Such difficult to treat and high risk patients were accrued to phase II studies with ANP [168]. The results are summarized in Table 5.

Recurrent, progressive multicentric gliomas (MCGs) have poor prognosis with no curative standard treatments available. Solitary low grade gliomas in children and adults were extensively studied and reviewed, but only a small number of reports were published on MCG [172-175]. For a solitary tumor, the prognosis improves with the extent of surgical resection, which does not apply to MCG. There was no difference in overall survival of patients not treated after surgery versus patients who underwent radiation therapy [172]. The overall survival was also not different for patients after radiation therapy or after radiation and chemotherapy with lomustine. In one of the studies of MCG with 11 patients, 8 patients were treated with different chemotherapy agents, 1 with radiation therapy, 1 with chemotherapy and radiation therapy, and 1 was not treated [173]. Two patients obtained remission of unspecified type, 5 had stabilization and 4 patients died. The other reports describe single cases or a small series without statistical data [172-176]. ANP was used in MCG in phase II trials and the results of the treatment in the first 12 children were already published [177] (Table 5).

Atypical teratoid/rhabdoid tumors (AT/RTs) are highly malignant but rare pediatric neoplasms. Standard treatment includes surgical resection followed by radiation therapy and chemotherapy [178, 179]. The responses to the standard therapy have been described, but unfortunately they are short-lasting and are followed by progression and patient death [178-181]. Typical feature of AT/RT is mutation of INI1 gene [111, 112]. INI1 arrests the cells at the G1-S checkpoint through induction of p16 and repression of transcription of cyclinD1 [114, 182]. Mutated INI protein dislocates from the nucleus to the cytoplasm where it remains inactive. ANP inhibits complex cyclin D1/CDK4 and cyclin E/CDK2 and interrupts INI1 transport from nucleus to cytoplasm, which results in inhibition of AT/RT growth [57, 58, 183].

Preliminary results of phase II studies of ANP and AT/RT have already been reported [114]. The group of 11 children was treated under study protocol. All patients underwent prior surgery, 5 were followed with radiation therapy, 9 with chemotherapy and developed progression of the disease, except for one non-evaluable case. In the group of 8 evaluable patients, there were 2 cases of CR, 1 PR, 1 SD and 4 cases of PD. Maximum survival was approximately 2 years from the start of ANP.

The data of preliminary results of clinical studies in high-risk pediatric brain tumor patients are summarized in Table 5.

Concluding Remarks and Perspectives

Rapidly expanding understanding of molecular biology of cancer cells resulted in an increasing number of targeted therapies in clinical investigations. The initial excitement, centered around imatinib and trastuzumab, raised hopes that difficult to treat primary brain tumors will also respond to a new generation of highly specific treatments. The development of currently used agents began at the time when scientists were interested in individual genes and signaling pathways, and resulted in the design of drugs oriented toward single targets. The hopes that such drugs will control extremely complex system represented by neoplastic cells are unrealistic [184, 185]. Neoplastic cells form an extremely complex and robust system which is maintained in the presence of serious perturbations [184]. Most of neoplastic characteristics arise from complex interactions which form a number of interrelated networks; for instance, signaling, protein-protein, transcription and metabolic networks [186]. In this respect, molecular interactions inside neoplastic cells can be compared to the internet. The networks are composed of nodes and links connecting them together. The most important nodes which regulate a large number of events form "hubs" [187]. Signaling network in human cells is extremely complex and consists of 1,543 types of receptors, 518 protein kinases, and close to 2,000 transcription factors [188-191]. The robustness of the neoplasm is assured by redundancy, feedback controls, modularity, structural stability, and gradual degradation of function in response to damage [184, 192]. These features help malignant cells escape from the control of the agents which are aimed at single targets. In this respect, imatinib was highly effective in the early stages of chronic myelogenous leukemia, but failed in the advanced stage [193]. Mutations in the *BCR-ABL* region are responsible for resistance to imatinib [194]. A higher success can be accomplished by designing the drugs targeting hubs of the network and multiple targets. Agents affecting multiple ERBB receptors (lapatinib, C1-1033, EKB-569) and ERBB and VEGFR (AEE788, EXEL 7647) may show higher clinical activity but their application may lead to unacceptable toxicity [22, 195]. On the other hand, a treatment using anti-ERBB agents in combination with mTOR may offer better results [196].

The ultimate success in controlling the neoplastic process would require elimination of neoplastic stem cells. Malignant stem cells have been identified in different human brain tumors [197-199]. The most promising targets in this area are Hh, MYC and Wnt pathways [200, 201]. Other important strategies include induction of apoptosis and cell cycle arrest through activation of *TP53* and *p21*. ANP explores multiple targets crucial in control of growth of brain tumors, including growth factor receptors (TGFBRI), signaling pathways (AKT/PTEN and RAS), cell cycle control (MYCC, p21, INI1) apoptosis, and cellular and nuclear transports, which gives this treatment a better chance for durable results.

Phase II studies of most of agents affecting single targets in primary brain tumors failed to show the results of clinical significance. The results of the treatment with erlotinib and imatinib with hydroxyurea are promising, but require confirmation by phase III studies [134, 135, 138, 139] . Combination therapy of bevacizumab and irinotecan contributed to a higher percentage of complete and partial responses, but was associated with significant toxicity. Clinical trials with multitargeted ANP in difficult to treat brain tumors, including recurrent and progressed GBM and DBSG resulted in favorable objective response rates, overall survival and progression free survival. The results of treatment of difficult to manage cases of PNET, multicentric glioma and AT/RT are encouraging, but will require confirmation in the larger population of patients. A low percentage of acute toxicity and no incidence of chronic toxicity allow administration of ANP for an extended period of time to assure proper control and prevention of tumor recurrence. Substantial data in this chapter are coming from meeting abstracts. Such data should be treated with caution until they pass the scrutiny of peer review. Dynamic expansion of the research on targeted therapies and identification of patients who are prospective responders promises the design and introduction of new agents of higher efficacy in the near future.

References

[1] Ehrlich P, in *Gesammelte Arbeiten,* Himmelweit F, Ed. (Springer-Verlag, Berlin, 1957).

[2] Burzynski SR. Clinical Application of Body Epigenetic System. Multi-Targeted Therapy for Primary Brain Tumors. *World and Ehrlich Conference on Dosing of Magic Bullets. September 9-11, 2004, Nürnberg, Germany.* 2004.

[3] Green MR. Targeting targeted therapy. *N Engl J Med* 2004;350:2191-3.

[4] Vogel CL, Cobleigh MA, Tripathy D, et al. Efficacy and safety of trastuzumab as a single agent in first-line treatment of HER2-overexpressing metastatic breast cancer. *J Clin Oncol* 2002;20:719-26.

[5] Kris MG, Natale RB, Herbst RS, et al. Efficacy of gefitinib, an inhibitor of the epidermal growth factor receptor tyrosine kinase, in symptomatic patients with non-small cell lung cancer: a randomized trial. *JAMA* 2003;290:2149-58.

[6] Giaccone G, Herbst RS, Manegold C, et al. Gefitinib in combination with gemcitabine and cisplatin in advanced non-small-cell lung cancer: a phase III trial--INTACT 1. *J Clin Oncol* 2004;22:777-84.

[7] Herbst RS, Giaccone G, Schiller JH, et al. Gefitinib in combination with paclitaxel and carboplatin in advanced non-small-cell lung cancer: a phase III trial--INTACT 2. *J Clin Oncol* 2004;22:785-94.

[8] Slamon DJ, Leyland-Jones B, Shak S, et al. Use of chemotherapy plus a monoclonal antibody against HER2 for metastatic breast cancer that overexpresses HER2. *N Engl J Med* 2001;344:783-92.

[9] DeAngelis LM. Chemotherapy for brain tumors--a new beginning. *N Engl J Med* 2005;352:1036-8.

[10] Stupp R, Mason WP, van den Bent MJ, et al. Radiotherapy plus concomitant and adjuvant temozolomide for glioblastoma. *N Engl J Med* 2005;352:987-96.

[11] Lashford LS, Thiesse P, Jouvet A, et al. Temozolomide in malignant gliomas of childhood: a United Kingdom Children's Cancer Study Group and French Society for Pediatric Oncology Intergroup Study. *J Clin Oncol* 2002;20:4684-91.

[12] Hegi ME, Diserens AC, Gorlia T, et al. MGMT gene silencing and benefit from temozolomide in glioblastoma. *N Engl J Med* 2005;352:997-1003.

[13] Fine HA, Figg WD, Jaeckle K, et al. Phase II trial of the antiangiogenic agent thalidomide in patients with recurrent high-grade gliomas. *J Clin Oncol* 2000;18:708-15.

[14] Baumann F, Bjeljac M, Kollias SS, et al. Combined thalidomide and temozolomide treatment in patients with glioblastoma multiforme. *J Neurooncol* 2004;67:191-200.

[15] Glass J. Phase I/II study of carboplatin and thalidomide in recurrent glioblastoma. *Proceedings of the American Society of Clinical Oncology. Abstract #551.* 1999.

[16] Goldman S, Tomita T, Marymont M, et al. Thalidomide and carboplatin in the treatment of brain stem glioma. *Neurooncol.* 2004;6:456.

[17] Cavaliere R, Farace E, Wen P, Schiff D. Thalidomide-associated thromboembolic events in patients with high-grade gliomas. *Neurooncol.* 2004;6:372.

[18] Fisher PG, Buffler PA. Malignant gliomas in 2005: where to GO from here? *JAMA* 2005;293:615-7.

[19] Zheng CJ, Han LY, Yap CW, Xie B, Chen YZ. Trends in exploration of therapeutic targets. *Drug News Perspect* 2005;18:109-27.

[20] Burzynski SR. The present state of antineoplaston research (1). *Integr Cancer Ther* 2004;3:47-58.

[21] Hynes NE, Lane HA. ERBB receptors and cancer: the complexity of targeted inhibitors. *Nat Rev Cancer* 2005;5:341-54.

[22] Newton HB. Molecular neuro-oncology and development of targeted therapeutic strategies for brain tumors. Part 1: Growth factor and Ras signaling pathways. *Expert Rev Anticancer Ther* 2003;3:595-614.

[23] Frederick L, Wang XY, Eley G, James CD. Diversity and frequency of epidermal growth factor receptor mutations in human glioblastomas. *Cancer Res* 2000;60:1383-7.

[24] Ekstrand AJ, Sugawa N, James CD, Collins VP. Amplified and rearranged epidermal growth factor receptor genes in human glioblastomas reveal deletions of sequences encoding portions of the N- and/or C-terminal tails. *Proc Natl Acad Sci U S A* 1992;89:4309-13.

[25] Hurtt MR, Moossy J, Donovan-Peluso M, Locker J. Amplification of epidermal growth factor receptor gene in gliomas: histopathology and prognosis. *J Neuropathol Exp Neurol* 1992;51:84-90.

[26] Nagane M, Levitzki A, Gazit A, Cavenee WK, Huang HJ. Drug resistance of human glioblastoma cells conferred by a tumor-specific mutant epidermal growth factor receptor through modulation of Bcl-XL and caspase-3-like proteases. *Proc Natl Acad Sci U S A* 1998;95:5724-9.

[27] Lal A, Glazer CA, Martinson HM, et al. Mutant epidermal growth factor receptor up-regulates molecular effectors of tumor invasion. *Cancer Res* 2002;62:3335-9.

[28] Muhsin M, Graham J, Kirkpatrick P. Gefitinib. *Nat Rev Drug Discov* 2003;2:515-6.

[29] Heimberger AB, Learn CA, Archer GE, et al. Brain tumors in mice are susceptible to blockade of epidermal growth factor receptor (EGFR) with the oral, specific, EGFR-tyrosine kinase inhibitor ZD1839 (iressa). *Clin Cancer Res* 2002;8:3496-502.

[30] Guillamo JS, Leuraud P, de Bouard S. Antiproliferative and anti-invasive EGFR amplification dependent and anti-angiogenic EGFR amplification independent activity

of ZD1839 (Iressa) tyrosine kinase inhibitor on human glioblastomas. *Proc. Am. Assoc. Cancer Res.* 2003;44:231.

[31] Dowell J, Minna JD, Kirkpatrick P. Erlotinib hydrochloride. *Nat Rev Drug Discov* 2005;4:13-4.

[32] Westermark B, Heldin CH, Nister M. Platelet-derived growth factor in human glioma. *Glia* 1995;15:257-63.

[33] Claesson-Welsh L. Platelet-derived growth factor receptor signals. *J Biol Chem* 1994;269:32023-6.

[34] Lokker NA, Sullivan CM, Hollenbach SJ, Israel MA, Giese NA. Platelet-derived growth factor (PDGF) autocrine signaling regulates survival and mitogenic pathways in glioblastoma cells: evidence that the novel PDGF-C and PDGF-D ligands may play a role in the development of brain tumors. *Cancer Res* 2002;62:3729-35.

[35] Richardson WD, Pringle N, Mosley MJ, Westermark B, Dubois-Dalcq M. A role for platelet-derived growth factor in normal gliogenesis in the central nervous system. *Cell* 1988;53:309-19.

[36] Guha A, Dashner K, Black PM, Wagner JA, Stiles CD. Expression of PDGF and PDGF receptors in human astrocytoma operation specimens supports the existence of an autocrine loop. *Int J Cancer* 1995;60:168-73.

[37] Hermanson M, Funa K, Hartman M, et al. Platelet-derived growth factor and its receptors in human glioma tissue: expression of messenger RNA and protein suggests the presence of autocrine and paracrine loops. *Cancer Res* 1992;52:3213-9.

[38] Savage DG, Antman KH. Imatinib mesylate--a new oral targeted therapy. *N Engl J Med* 2002;346:683-93.

[39] Kilic T, Alberta JA, Zdunek PR, et al. Intracranial inhibition of platelet-derived growth factor-mediated glioblastoma cell growth by an orally active kinase inhibitor of the 2-phenylaminopyrimidine class. *Cancer Res* 2000;60:5143-50.

[40] Sawyers CL. Opportunities and challenges in the development of kinase inhibitor therapy for cancer. *Genes Dev* 2003;17:2998-3010.

[41] Hanahan D, Folkman J. Patterns and emerging mechanisms of the angiogenic switch during tumorigenesis. *Cell* 1996;86:353-64.

[42] Ferrara N, Gerber HP, LeCouter J. The biology of VEGF and its receptors. *Nat Med* 2003;9:669-76.

[43] Veikkola T, Karkkainen M, Claesson-Welsh L, Alitalo K. Regulation of angiogenesis via vascular endothelial growth factor receptors. *Cancer Res* 2000;60:203-12.

[44] Komarova NL, Sengupta A, Nowak MA. Mutation-selection networks of cancer initiation: tumor suppressor genes and chromosomal instability. *J Theor Biol* 2003;223:433-50.

[45] Ellis LM. Bevacizumab. *Nat Rev Drug Discov* 2005;Suppl:S8-9.

[46] Siegel PM, Massague J. Cytostatic and apoptotic actions of TGF-beta in homeostasis and cancer. *Nat Rev Cancer* 2003;3:807-21.

[47] Grady WM. Transforming growth factor-beta, Smads, and cancer. *Clin Cancer Res* 2005;11:3151-4.

[48] Downing JR. TGF-beta signaling, tumor suppression, and acute lymphoblastic leukemia. *N Engl J Med* 2004;351:528-30.

[49] Derynck R, Akhurst RJ, Balmain A. TGF-beta signaling in tumor suppression and cancer progression. *Nat Genet* 2001;29:117-29.

[50] Bhowmick NA, Ghiassi M, Bakin A, et al. Transforming growth factor-beta1 mediates epithelial to mesenchymal transdifferentiation through a RhoA-dependent mechanism. *Mol Biol Cell* 2001;12:27-36.

[51] Platten M, Wick W, Weller M. Malignant glioma biology: role for TGF-beta in growth, motility, angiogenesis, and immune escape. *Microsc Res Tech* 2001;52:401-10.

[52] Jennings MT, Maciunas RJ, Carver R, et al. TGF beta 1 and TGF beta 2 are potential growth regulators for low-grade and malignant gliomas in vitro: evidence in support of an autocrine hypothesis. *Int J Cancer* 1991;49:129-39.

[53] Isoe S, Naganuma H, Nakano S, et al. Resistance to growth inhibition by transforming growth factor-beta in malignant glioma cells with functional receptors. *J Neurosurg* 1998;88:529-34.

[54] Kjellman C, Olofsson SP, Hansson O, et al. Expression of TGF-beta isoforms, TGF-beta receptors, and SMAD molecules at different stages of human glioma. *Int J Cancer* 2000;89:251-8.

[55] Li DM, Sun H. TEP1, encoded by a candidate tumor suppressor locus, is a novel protein tyrosine phosphatase regulated by transforming growth factor beta. *Cancer Res* 1997;57:2124-9.

[56] Liau LM, Fakhrai H, Black KL. Prolonged survival of rats with intracranial C6 gliomas by treatment with TGF-beta antisense gene. *Neurol Res* 1998;20:742-7.

[57] Waldbillig R, Burzynski SR. Mechanism of action, uptake, and gene array studies on the antineoplastic agent phenylacetylglutamine (PG) in human glioma cells U-87. *Neuro-oncol* 2003;5:309.

[58] Waldbillig RJ, Patil S, Burzynski SR. Uptake and intracellular binding of the antineoplastic agents phenylacetic acid and phenylacetylglutamine (PG): effects on epigenetic mechanisms of gene regulation and gene expression. Report to FDA. 2004.

[59] Malumbres M, Barbacid M. RAS oncogenes: the first 30 years. *Nat Rev Cancer* 2003;3:459-65.

[60] Adjei AA. Blocking oncogenic Ras signaling for cancer therapy. *J Natl Cancer Inst* 2001;93:1062-74.

[61] Bos JL. ras oncogenes in human cancer: a review. *Cancer Res* 1989;49:4682-9.

[62] Meder D, Simons K. Cell biology. Ras on the roundabout. *Science* 2005;307:1731-3.

[63] Rocks O, Peyker A, Kahms M, et al. An acylation cycle regulates localization and activity of palmitoylated Ras isoforms. *Science* 2005;307:1746-52.

[64] Chiu VK, Bivona T, Hach A, et al. Ras signalling on the endoplasmic reticulum and the Golgi. *Nat Cell Biol* 2002;4:343-50.

[65] Cichowski K, Jacks T. NF1 tumor suppressor gene function: narrowing the GAP. *Cell* 2001;104:593-604.

[66] Newton HB. Molecular neuro-oncology and development of targeted therapeutic strategies for brain tumors. Part 2: PI3K/Akt/PTEN, mTOR, SHH/PTCH and angiogenesis. *Expert Rev Anticancer Ther* 2004;4:105-28.

[67] Guha A, Feldkamp MM, Lau N, Boss G, Pawson A. Proliferation of human malignant astrocytomas is dependent on Ras activation. *Oncogene* 1997;15:2755-65.

[68] Mazieres J, Pradines A, Favre G. Perspectives on farnesyl transferase inhibitors in cancer therapy. *Cancer Lett* 2004;206:159-67.

[69] Gotlib J. Farnesyltransferase inhibitor therapy in acute myelogenous leukemia. *Curr Hematol Rep* 2005;4:77-84.

[70] Winter-Vann AM, Casey PJ. Post-prenylation-processing enzymes as new targets in oncogenesis. *Nat Rev Cancer* 2005;5:405-12.

[71] Whyte DB, Kirschmeier P, Hockenberry TN, et al. K- and N-Ras are geranylgeranylated in cells treated with farnesyl protein transferase inhibitors. *J Biol Chem* 1997;272:14459-64.

[72] Sebti SM, Der CJ. Opinion: Searching for the elusive targets of farnesyltransferase inhibitors. *Nat Rev Cancer* 2003;3:945-51.

[73] Shack S, Chen LC, Miller AC, Danesi R, Samid D. Increased susceptibility of ras-transformed cells to phenylacetate is associated with inhibition of p21ras isoprenylation and phenotypic reversion. *Int J Cancer* 1995;63:124-9.

[74] Fujii T, Nakamura AM, Yokoyama G, et al. Antineoplaston induces G_1 arrest by PKCalpha and MAPK pathway in SKBR-3 breast cancer cells. *Oncol Rep* 2005;14:489-94.

[75] Vivanco I, Sawyers CL. The phosphatidylinositol 3-Kinase AKT pathway in human cancer. *Nat Rev Cancer* 2002;2:489-501.

[76] Bjornsti MA, Houghton PJ. The TOR pathway: a target for cancer therapy. *Nat Rev Cancer* 2004;4:335-48.

[77] Sonoda Y, Ozawa T, Aldape KD, et al. Akt pathway activation converts anaplastic astrocytoma to glioblastoma multiforme in a human astrocyte model of glioma. *Cancer Res* 2001;61:6674-8.

[78] Ramaswamy S, Nakamura N, Vazquez F, et al. Regulation of G1 progression by the PTEN tumor suppressor protein is linked to inhibition of the phosphatidylinositol 3-kinase/Akt pathway. *Proc Natl Acad Sci U S A* 1999;96:2110-5.

[79] Mills GB, Lu Y, Kohn EC. Linking molecular therapeutics to molecular diagnostics: inhibition of the FRAP/RAFT/TOR component of the PI3K pathway preferentially blocks PTEN mutant cells in vitro and in vivo. *Proc Natl Acad Sci U S A* 2001;98:10031-3.

[80] Massague J. G1 cell-cycle control and cancer. *Nature* 2004;432:298-306.

[81] Burzynski SR, Weaver RA, Janicki T, et al. Long-term Survival of High-Risk Pediatric Patients With Primitive Neuroectodermal Tumors Treated With Antineoplastons A10 and AS2-1. *Integr Cancer Ther* 2005;4:168-77.

[82] Pelengaris S, Khan M, Evan G. c-MYC: more than just a matter of life and death. *Nat Rev Cancer* 2002;2:764-76.

[83] Bachireddy P, Bendapudi PK, Felsher DW. Getting at MYC through RAS. *Clin Cancer Res* 2005;11:4278-81.

[84] Sears R, Nuckolls F, Haura E, et al. Multiple Ras-dependent phosphorylation pathways regulate Myc protein stability. *Genes Dev* 2000;14:2501-14.

[85] Downward J. Targeting RAS signalling pathways in cancer therapy. *Nat Rev Cancer* 2003;3:11-22.

[86] Perez-Roger I, Kim SH, Griffiths B, Sewing A, Land H. Cyclins D1 and D2 mediate myc-induced proliferation via sequestration of p27(Kip1) and p21(Cip1). *Embo J* 1999;18:5310-20.

[87] O'Hagan RC, Ohh M, David G, et al. Myc-enhanced expression of Cul1 promotes ubiquitin-dependent proteolysis and cell cycle progression. *Genes Dev* 2000;14:2185-91.

[88] Murray AW. Recycling the cell cycle: cyclins revisited. *Cell* 2004;116:221-34.

[89] Stevaux O, Dyson NJ. A revised picture of the E2F transcriptional network and RB function. *Curr Opin Cell Biol* 2002;14:684-91.

[90] Sherr CJ, Roberts JM. CDK inhibitors: positive and negative regulators of G1-phase progression. *Genes Dev* 1999;13:1501-12.

[91] Staller P, Peukert K, Kiermaier A, et al. Repression of p15INK4b expression by Myc through association with Miz-1. *Nat Cell Biol* 2001;3:392-9.

[92] Sears RC, Nevins JR. Signaling networks that link cell proliferation and cell fate. *J Biol Chem* 2002;277:11617-20.

[93] Gorospe M, Shack S, Guyton KZ, Samid D, Holbrook NJ. Up-regulation and functional role of p21Waf1/Cip1 during growth arrest of human breast carcinoma MCF-7 cells by phenylacetate. *Cell Growth Differ* 1996;7:1609-15.

[94] Brown JM, Attardi LD. The role of apoptosis in cancer development and treatment response. *Nat Rev Cancer* 2005;5:231-7.

[95] Broker LE, Kruyt FA, Giaccone G. Cell death independent of caspases: a review. *Clin Cancer Res* 2005;11:3155-62.

[96] Fennell DA. Caspase regulation in non-small cell lung cancer and its potential for therapeutic exploitation. *Clin Cancer Res* 2005;11:2097-105.

[97] Schimmer AD. Inhibitor of apoptosis proteins: translating basic knowledge into clinical practice. *Cancer Res* 2004;64:7183-90.

[98] Ghobrial IM, Witzig TE, Adjei AA. Targeting apoptosis pathways in cancer therapy. *CA Cancer J Clin* 2005;55:178-94.

[99] Hueber AO, Zornig M, Lyon D, et al. Requirement for the CD95 receptor-ligand pathway in c-Myc-induced apoptosis. *Science* 1997;278:1305-9.

[100] Lutz W, Fulda S, Jeremias I, Debatin KM, Schwab M. MycN and IFNgamma cooperate in apoptosis of human neuroblastoma cells. *Oncogene* 1998;17:339-46.

[101] Klefstrom J, Vastrik I, Saksela E, et al. c-Myc induces cellular susceptibility to the cytotoxic action of TNF-alpha. *Embo J* 1994;13:5442-50.

[102] Hockenbery D, Nunez G, Milliman C, Schreiber RD, Korsmeyer SJ. Bcl-2 is an inner mitochondrial membrane protein that blocks programmed cell death. *Nature* 1990;348:334-6.

[103] Levine AJ. p53, the cellular gatekeeper for growth and division. *Cell* 1997;88:323-31.

[104] el-Deiry WS, Harper JW, O'Connor PM, et al. WAF1/CIP1 is induced in p53-mediated G1 arrest and apoptosis. *Cancer Res* 1994;54:1169-74.

[105] Yu J, Zhang L, Hwang PM, et al. Identification and classification of p53-regulated genes. *Proc Natl Acad Sci U S A* 1999;96:14517-22.

[106] Clarke AR, Gledhill S, Hooper ML, Bird CC, Wyllie AH. p53 dependence of early apoptotic and proliferative responses within the mouse intestinal epithelium following gamma-irradiation. *Oncogene* 1994;9:1767-73.

[107] Lozano G, Zambetti GP. What have animal models taught us about the p53 pathway? *J Pathol* 2005;205:206-20.

[108] Liu L, Samid D. Mutant p53 as a target of phenylacetate in human glioblastoma. *Presented at the 8th Annual Meeting of the American Association for Cancer Research.* March 1995, Toronto, Canada.

[109] Adam L, Crepin M, Savin C, Israel L. Sodium phenylacetate induces growth inhibition and Bcl-2 down-regulation and apoptosis in MCF7ras cells in vitro and in nude mice. *Cancer Res* 1995;55:5156-60.

[110] Adam L, Crepin M, Israel L. Tumor growth inhibition, apoptosis, and Bcl-2 down-regulation of MCF-7ras tumors by sodium phenylacetate and tamoxifen combination. *Cancer Res* 1997;57:1023-9.

[111] Biegel JA, Tan L, Zhang F, et al. Alterations of the hSNF5/INI1 gene in central nervous system atypical teratoid/rhabdoid tumors and renal and extrarenal rhabdoid tumors. *Clin Cancer Res* 2002;8:3461-7.

[112] Versteege I, Medjkane S, Rouillard D, Delattre O. A key role of the hSNF5/INI1 tumour suppressor in the control of the G1-S transition of the cell cycle. *Oncogene* 2002;21:6403-12.

[113] Kau TR, Way JC, Silver PA. Nuclear transport and cancer: from mechanism to intervention. *Nat Rev Cancer* 2004;4:106-17.

[114] Burzynski SR, Weaver R, Bestak M, et al. Phase II studies of antineoplastons A10 and AS2-1 in children with atypical teratoid/rhabdoid tumors of the central nervous system. A preliminary report. *Neurooncol.* 2004;6:427.

[115] Liau MC, Liau CP, Burzynski SR. Potentiation of induced terminal differentiation by phenylacetic acid and related chemicals. *Int J Exptl Clin Chemother* 1992;5:9-17.

[116] Zardo G, Tiirikainen MI, Hong C, et al. Integrated genomic and epigenomic analyses pinpoint biallelic gene inactivation in tumors. *Nat Genet* 2002;32:453-8.

[117] Costello JF, Berger MS, Huang HS, Cavenee WK. Silencing of p16/CDKN2 expression in human gliomas by methylation and chromatin condensation. *Cancer Res* 1996;56:2405-10.

[118] Bachman KE, Herman JG, Corn PG, et al. Methylation-associated silencing of the tissue inhibitor of metalloproteinase-3 gene suggest a suppressor role in kidney, brain, and other human cancers. *Cancer Res* 1999;59:798-802.

[119] Feinberg AP, Tycko B. The history of cancer epigenetics. *Nat Rev Cancer* 2004;4:143-53.

[120] Ehrlich M. DNA methylation in cancer: too much, but also too little. *Oncogene* 2002;21:5400-13.

[121] Nishigaki M, Aoyagi K, Danjoh I, et al. Discovery of aberrant expression of R-RAS by cancer-linked DNA hypomethylation in gastric cancer using microarrays. *Cancer Res* 2005;65:2115-24.

[122] Jaenisch R, Bird A. Epigenetic regulation of gene expression: how the genome integrates intrinsic and environmental signals. *Nat Genet* 2003;33 Suppl:245-54.

[123] Ringrose L, Paro R. Epigenetic regulation of cellular memory by the Polycomb and Trithorax group proteins. *Annu Rev Genet* 2004;38:413-43.

[124] Issa JP, Kantarjian H. Azacitidine. *Nat Rev Drug Discov* 2005;Suppl:S6-7.

[125] Central Brain Tumor Registry of the United States (CBTRUS). 2004-2005 Primary Brain Tumors in the United States Statistical Report, Years Data Collected 1997-2001.

[126] DeAngelis LM. Brain tumors. *N Engl J Med* 2001;344:114-23.

[127] Brada M, Thomas DGT, Bleehen NM, et al. Medical Research Council (MRC) randomized trial of adjuvant chemotherapy in high grade glioma (HGG) -- BRO5. *Proceedings of the American Society of Clinical Oncology. Abstract #1543.* 1998.

[128] Chamberlain MC, Kormanik PA. Practical guidelines for the treatment of malignant gliomas. *West J Med* 1998;168:114-20.

[129] Stevens MF, Hickman JA, Langdon SP, et al. Antitumor activity and pharmacokinetics in mice of 8-carbamoyl-3-methyl-imidazo[5,1-d]-1,2,3,5-tetrazin-4(3H)-one (CCRG 81045; M and B 39831), a novel drug with potential as an alternative to dacarbazine. *Cancer Res* 1987;47:5846-52.

[130] Newlands ES, Blackledge GR, Slack JA, et al. Phase I trial of temozolomide (CCRG 81045: M and B 39831: NSC 362856). *Br J Cancer* 1992;65:287-91.

[131] Yung WK, Albright RE, Olson J, et al. A phase II study of temozolomide vs. procarbazine in patients with glioblastoma multiforme at first relapse. *Br J Cancer* 2000;83:588-93.

[132] Wen PY, Yung WKA, Lamborn K, et al. Phase I/II study of imatinib mesylate (ST1571) for patients with recurrent malignant gliomas (NABTC 99-08). *Neurooncol.* 2004;6:385.

[133] van den Bent MJ, Brandes AA, van Oosterom A, et al. Multicentre phase II study of imatinib mesylate (Gleevec) in patients with recurrent glioblastoma: an EORTC NDDG/BTG intergroup study. *Neurooncol.* 2004;6:383.

[134] Dresemann G. Imatinib (STI 571)/ plus hydroxyurea: Safety and efficacy in pre-treated, progresive Glioblastoma Multiforme (GBM) patients (pts): An update on the initial 30 pts. *Proceedings of the American Society of Clinical Oncology. Abstract #1515.* 2005

[135] Reardon D, Quinn J, Rich J, et al. Imatinib mesylate (Gleevec) plus hydroxyurea: an effective regimen in the treatment of recurrent malignant glioma: phase 2 study results. *Neurooncol.* 2005;7:291.

[136] Rich JN, Reardon DA, Peery T, et al. Phase II trial of gefitinib in recurrent glioblastoma. *J Clin Oncol* 2004;22:133-42.

[137] Franceschi E, Lonardi S, Tosoni A, et al. Gefinitib (ZD1839) treatment for adult patients with progressive high-grade gliomas (HGG): An open label, single-arm, phase II study of the Gruppo Italiano Cooperative di Neuro-Oncologia (GICNO). *Proceedings of the American Society of Clinical Oncology. Abstract #2564.* 2005.

[138] Vogelbaum MA, Peereboom D, Stevens GHJ, Barnett GH, Brewer C. Response rate to single agent therapy with the EGFR tyrosine kinase inhibitor erlotinib in recurrent glioblastoma multiforme: results of a phase II study. *Neurooncol.* 2004;6:384.

[139] Cloughesy T, Yung A, Vrendenberg J, et al. Phase II study of erlotinib in recurrent GBM: Molecular predictors of outcome. *Proceedings of the American Society of Clinical Oncology. Abstract #1507.* 2005.

[140] Stark-Vance V. Bevacizumab and CPT-11 in the Treatment of Relapsed Malignant Glioma. *Neurooncol.* 2005;7:369.

[141] Gilbert M, Hess K, Liu V, et al. A phase 2 study of temozolomide (TMZ) and the farnesyltransferase inhibitor (FTI) lonafarnib (sarazartm, SCH66336) in recurrent glioblastoma. *Neurooncol* 2005; 7:401.

[142] Galanis E, Buckner JC, Maurer MJ, et al. N997B: Phase II trial of CCI-779 in recurrent glioblastoma multiforme (GBM): Updated results and correlative laboratory analysis. *Proceedings of the American Society of Clinical Oncology. Abstract #1515.* 2005.

[143] Fine HA, Kim L, Royce C, et al. Results from phase II trial of enzastaurin (LY317615) in patients with recurrent high grade gliomas. *Proceedings of the American Society of Clinical Oncology. Abstract #1504.* 2005.

[144] Weaver RA, Burzynski SR, Bestak M. Phase II study of antineoplastons A10 and AS2-1 (ANP) in recurrent glioblastoma multiforme. *Neurooncol.* 2004;6:384.

[145] Weaver RA, Burzynski SR, Janicki T, Burzynski B. Long-term survival in patients with glioblastoma multiforme treated in phase II studies with ANP. *Neurooncol.* 2005;7:799.

[146] Smith MA, Freidlin B, Ries LA, Simon R. Trends in reported incidence of primary malignant brain tumors in children in the United States. *J Natl Cancer Inst* 1998;90:1269-77.

[147] Guillamo JS, Doz F, Delattre JY. Brain stem gliomas. *Curr Opin Neurol* 2001;14:711-5.

[148] Freeman CR, Farmer JP. Pediatric brain stem gliomas: a review. *Int J Radiat Oncol Biol Phys* 1998;40:265-71.

[149] Gilbertson RJ, Hill DA, Hernan R, et al. ERBB1 is amplified and overexpressed in high-grade diffusely infiltrative pediatric brain stem glioma. *Clin Cancer Res* 2003;9:3620-4.

[150] Louis DN, Rubio MP, Correa KM, Gusella JF, von Deimling A. Molecular genetics of pediatric brain stem gliomas. Application of PCR techniques to small and archival brain tumor specimens. *J Neuropathol Exp Neurol* 1993;52:507-15.

[151] Cheng Y, Ng HK, Zhang SF, et al. Genetic alterations in pediatric high-grade astrocytomas. *Hum Pathol* 1999;30:1284-90.

[152] Mandell LR, Kadota R, Freeman C, et al. There is no role for hyperfractionated radiotherapy in the management of children with newly diagnosed diffuse intrinsic brainstem tumors: results of a Pediatric Oncology Group phase III trial comparing conventional vs. hyperfractionated radiotherapy. *Int J Radiat Oncol Biol Phys* 1999;43:959-64.

[153] Freeman CR, Kepner J, Kun LE, et al. A detrimental effect of a combined chemotherapy-radiotherapy approach in children with diffuse intrinsic brain stem gliomas? *Int J Radiat Oncol Biol Phys* 2000;47:561-4.

[154] Allen J, Siffert J, Donahue B, et al. A phase I/II study of carboplatin combined with hyperfractionated radiotherapy for brainstem gliomas. *Cancer* 1999;86:1064-9.

[155] Freeman CR, Perilongo G. Chemotherapy for brain stem gliomas. *Childs Nerv Syst* 1999;15:545-53.

[156] Bouffet E, Raquin M, Doz F, et al. Radiotherapy followed by high dose busulfan and thiotepa: a prospective assessment of high dose chemotherapy in children with diffuse pontine gliomas. *Cancer* 2000;88:685-92.

[157] Broniscer A, Leite CC, Lanchote VL, Machado TM, Cristofani LM. Radiation therapy and high-dose tamoxifen in the treatment of patients with diffuse brainstem gliomas: results of a Brazilian cooperative study. Brainstem Glioma Cooperative Group. *J Clin Oncol* 2000;18:1246-53.

[158] Jennings MT, Sposto R, Boyett JM, et al. Preradiation chemotherapy in primary high-risk brainstem tumors: phase II study CCG-9941 of the Children's Cancer Group. *J Clin Oncol* 2002;20:3431-7.

[159] Doz F, Neuenschwander S, Bouffet E, et al. Carboplatin before and during radiation therapy for the treatment of malignant brain stem tumours: a study by the Societe Francaise d'Oncologie Pediatrique. *Eur J Cancer* 2002;38:815-9.

[160] Wolff JE, Westphal S, Molenkamp G, et al. Treatment of paediatric pontine glioma with oral trophosphamide and etoposide. *Br J Cancer* 2002;87:945-9.

[161] Massimino M, Gandola L, Spreafico F, et al. Intrinsic Brain Stem Tumor: Changing Strategies, Changing Results? *Neurooncol.* 2003;5:51.

[162] Broniscer A, Gajjar A. Supratentorial high-grade astrocytoma and diffuse brainstem glioma: two challenges for the pediatric oncologist. *Oncologist* 2004;9:197-206.

[163] Burzynski SR, Lewy RI, Weaver RA, et al. Phase II study of antineoplaston A10 and AS2-1 in patients with recurrent diffuse intrinsic brain stem glioma: a preliminary report. *Drugs R D* 2003;4:91-101.

[164] Burzynski SR, Lewy RI, Weaver R, et al. Long-term survival and complete response of a patient with recurrent diffuse intrinsic brain stem glioblastoma multiforme. *Integr Cancer Ther* 2004;3:257-61.

[165] Burzynski SR, Weaver RA, Janicki T. Long-term survival in phase II studies of Antineoplastons A10 and AS2-1 (ANP) in patients with diffuse intrinsic brain stem glioma. *Neurooncol* 2004;6:386.

[166] Burzynski SR, Janicki TJ, Weaver RA, Burzynski B. Targeted therapy with antineoplastons A10 and AS2-1 (ANP) of high grade recurrent and progressive brain stem gliomas. *Presented at the 16th International Congress on Anti-Cancer Treatment. Paris, France. February 1-4.* 2005.

[167] Burzynski SR, Weaver RA, Janicki TJ, Burzynski B, Jurida GF. Targeted therapy with ANP in children less than 4 years old with inoperable brain stem gliomas. *Neurooncol.* 2005;7:300.

[168] Burzynski SR, Weaver RA, Janicki T, et al. Long-term Survival of High-Risk Pediatric Patients With Primitive Neuroectodermal Tumors Treated With Antineoplastons A10 and AS2-1. *Integr Cancer Ther* 2005;4:168-77.

[169] Taylor RE, Bailey CC, Robinson K, et al. Results of a randomized study of preradiation chemotherapy versus radiotherapy alone for nonmetastatic medulloblastoma: The International Society of Paediatric Oncology/United Kingdom Children's Cancer Study Group PNET-3 Study. *J Clin Oncol* 2003;21:1581-91.

[170] Gajjar A, Hernan R, Kocak M, et al. Clinical, histopathologic, and molecular markers of prognosis: toward a new disease risk stratification system for medulloblastoma. *J Clin Oncol* 2004;22:984-93.

[171] Fisher PG, Burger PC, Eberhart CG. Biologic risk stratification of medulloblastoma: the real time is now. *J Clin Oncol* 2004;22:971-4.

[172] Chamberlain MC, Grafe MR. Recurrent chiasmatic-hypothalamic glioma treated with oral etoposide. *J Clin Oncol* 1995;13:2072-6.

[173] Mamelak AN, Prados MD, Obana WG, Cogen PH, Edwards MS. Treatment options and prognosis for multicentric juvenile pilocytic astrocytoma. *J Neurosurg* 1994;81:24-30.

[174] Zamponi N, Rychlicki F, Ducati A, et al. Multicentric glioma with unusual clinical presentation. *Childs Nerv Syst* 2001;17:101-5.

[175] Shaw EG, Wisoff JH. Prospective clinical trials of intracranial low-grade glioma in adults and children. *Neurooncol* 2003;5:153-60.

[176] Sim KB, Hong SK. Multicentric juvenile pilocytic astrocytoma occurring primarily in the trigone of the lateral ventricle. *Childs Nerv Syst* 1999;15:477-81.

[177] Burzynski SR, Weaver RA, Lewy RI, et al. Phase II study of antineoplaston A10 and AS2-1 in children with recurrent and progressive multicentric glioma: a preliminary report. *Drugs R D* 2004;5:315-26.

[178] Lafrancois, M.A., Scott, M., Goumnerova, L., Proctor, M., Marcus, K., Pomeroy, S., Chordas, C., Turner, C., and Kieran, M. Sustained remission after recurrent central nervous system atypical teratoid/rhabdoid tumor: a report of two cases. *Neurooncol.* 2003; 5: 50.

[179] Janss, A.J., Changhu, C., Shu, H., Fisher, M., Belasco, J., Rorke, L.B., Biegel, J., Phillips, P.C. Atypical teratoid rhaboid tumors (AT/RT) of the central nervous system (CNS): Survival and treatment response in 35 patients diagnosed at Children's Hospital of Philadelphia. *Neurooncol.* 2004;6:459.

[180] Dreyer ZE, Kadota RP, Stewart CF, et al. Phase 2 study of idarubicin in pediatric brain tumors: Pediatric Oncology Group study POG 9237. *Neurooncol.* 2003;5:261-7.

[181] Strother LD, Burger P, Aronin P, et al. Outcome of therapy for atypical teratoid/rhabdoid tumors (ATRT) on pediatric oncology group study (POG) 9233/34. *Neurooncol.* 2004;6:466.

[182] Betz BL, Strobeck MW, Reisman DN, Knudsen ES, Weissman BE. Re-expression of hSNF5/INI1/BAF47 in pediatric tumor cells leads to G1 arrest associated with induction of p16ink4a and activation of RB. *Oncogene* 2002;21:5193-203.

[183] Zhang ZK, Davies KP, Allen J, et al. Cell cycle arrest and repression of cyclin D1 transcription by INI1/hSNF5. *Mol Cell Biol* 2002;22:5975-88.

[184] Kitano H. Cancer as a robust system: implications for anticancer therapy. *Nat Rev Cancer* 2004;4:227-35.

[185] Sawyers C. Targeted cancer therapy. *Nature* 2004;432:294-7.

[186] Barabasi AL, Oltvai ZN. Network biology: understanding the cell's functional organization. *Nat Rev Genet* 2004;5:101-13.

[187] Luscombe NM, Babu MM, Yu H, et al. Genomic analysis of regulatory network dynamics reveals large topological changes. *Nature* 2004;431:308-12.

[188] Papin JA, Hunter T, Palsson BO, Subramaniam S. Reconstruction of cellular signalling networks and analysis of their properties. *Nat Rev Mol Cell Biol* 2005;6:99-111.

[189] Venter JC, Adams MD, Myers EW, et al. The sequence of the human genome. *Science* 2001;291:1304-51.

[190] Manning G, Whyte DB, Martinez R, Hunter T, Sudarsanam S. The protein kinase complement of the human genome. *Science* 2002;298:1912-34.

[191] Lander ES, Linton LM, Birren B, et al. Initial sequencing and analysis of the human genome. *Nature* 2001;409:860-921.

[192] Kitano H. Cancer robustness: tumour tactics. *Nature* 2003;426:125.

[193] Hochhaus A. Cytogenetic and molecular mechanisms of resistance to imatinib. *Semin Hematol* 2003;40:69-79.

[194] Gorre ME, Mohammed M, Ellwood K, et al. Clinical resistance to STI-571 cancer therapy caused by *BCR-ABL* gene mutation or amplification. *Science* 2001;293:876-80.

[195] Traxler P, Allegrini PR, Brandt R, et al. AEE788: a dual family epidermal growth factor receptor/ErbB2 and vascular endothelial growth factor receptor tyrosine kinase inhibitor with antitumor and antiangiogenic activity. *Cancer Res* 2004;64:4931-41.

[196] Zhou X, Tan M, Stone Hawthorne V, et al. Activation of the Akt/mammalian target of rapamycin/4E-BP1 pathway by ErbB2 overexpression predicts tumor progression in breast cancers. *Clin Cancer Res* 2004;10:6779-88.

[197] Hemmati HD, Nakano I, Lazareff JA, et al. Cancerous stem cells can arise from pediatric brain tumors. *Proc Natl Acad Sci U S A* 2003;100:15178-83.

[198] Singh SK, Clarke ID, Terasaki M, et al. Identification of a cancer stem cell in human brain tumors. *Cancer Res* 2003;63:5821-8.

[199] Kondo T, Setoguchi T, Taga T. Persistence of a small subpopulation of cancer stem-like cells in the C6 glioma cell line. *Proc Natl Acad Sci U S A* 2004;101:781-6.

[200] Beachy PA, Karhadkar SS, Berman DM. Tissue repair and stem cell renewal in carcinogenesis. *Nature* 2004;432:324-31.

[201] Jain M, Arvanitis C, Chu K, et al. Sustained loss of a neoplastic phenotype by brief inactivation of MYC. *Science* 2002;297:102-4.

In: Brain Cancer Therapy and Surgical Interventions... ISBN 1-59454-974-5
Editor: Andrew V. Yang, pp. 113-125

Chapter V

Gamma Knife Radiosurgery for Metastatic Brain Tumors

***T. Shuto*[1]*, H. Fujino*[1]*, S. Inomori*[1] *and H. Nagano*[2]**
Departments of [1]Neurosurgery and [2]Radiation Oncology,
Yokohama Rosai Hospital, Yokohama, Kanagawa, Japan

Abstract

The development of cancer treatments with better outcomes and longer survival times continues to increase the chance of encountering metastatic brain tumors. Tumor removal by craniotomy and adjuvant whole brain radiotherapy (WBRT) are common methods of treatment, and stereotactic radiosurgery such as gamma knife radiosurgery (GKS) has recently become widely used. The major advantages of GKS are low invasiveness, short duration of hospitalization, effect independent of tumor histology, and repeatability. Deep-seated lesions in locations such as the brain stem are also good candidates for GKS. In addition, GKS is effective against metastatic brain tumors from radioresistant cancers such as renal cell carcinoma or malignant melanoma. Although good tumor growth control rate and low incidence of local recurrence have been reported, there is no prophylactic effect against the further development of new tumors. This disadvantage is overcome by the repeatability of GKS, which can be used to treat newly developed metastases following the first GKS. The optimum treatment for multiple metastatic brain tumors remains controversial. WBRT is standard, but more than 10-20 metastases can only be treated by GKS if the tumor diameters are less than 1 cm. On the other hand, WBRT is still important in the strategy for numerous metastases or metastatic cerebrospinal dissemination. Median survival time of patients who received GKS for metastatic brain tumors is less than 1 year, and more than 70% of patients died of systemic progression of the primary malignancy, not the brain metastases. Therefore, the goal of treatment by GKS is to avoid neurogenic death and to maintain good activity in daily life, not to achieve longer survival time. Radiosurgery should be considered as the optimum treatment modality for patients with brain metastases if the primary or distant metastases are well controlled, even if the lesions are multiple or newly developed after initial GKS.

Key-words: Metastatic brain tumor, radiosurgery, gamma knife, whole brain radiotherapy

Introduction

Nearly half of all patients with cancer will develop brain metastases [43], and the development of cancer treatments with improved outcomes and longer survival times continues to increase the chance of encountering metastatic brain tumors. Tumor removal by craniotomy and adjuvant whole brain radiotherapy (WBRT) are the most common methods of treatment [3, 18, 30, 39-41, 46], but stereotactic radiosurgery has recently become widely used [13, 14, 31, 64]. Gamma knife radiosurgery (GKS) has dramatically transformed the treatment strategy for metastatic brain tumors. This chapter reviews the advantages and disadvantages of GKS, and discusses the role of GKS in the current therapeutic strategy for metastatic brain tumors.

GKS: General Considerations

GKS can be performed under local anesthesia and causes minimum invasiveness. GKS uses the Leksell gamma unit (model B; Elekta Instruments, Inc.) and the treatment planning is undertaken with Gamma Plan software (Elekta). The Leksell frame is usually fixed with 4 point screw fixation. For patients with bone defects following frontal craniotomy, 3 point fixation or 4 point with cheek fixation at the side of the craniotomy is also available. After fixation of the Leksell frame, magnetic resonance (MR) images with gadolinium-diethylenetriaminepenta-acetic acid are obtained with 2 mm slices. Either delayed imaging after injection of the standard contrast dose or higher contrast dose is recommended to evaluate small brain metastases [72]. The MR images are transmitted via a network to the Gamma Plan treatment software.

After precise definition of the target (metastatic brain tumor), treatment planning is established using 4 types of collimator (4, 8, 14, 18 mm). Even an irregular tumor margin can be covered precisely using the multi-isocenter technique. Then, the appropriate delivered peripheral dose is decided depending mainly on the tumor volume and surrounding structures. The treatment is finished within a few hours in most cases, and the patient is discharged home the day after treatment. Therefore, the duration of hospitalization is only 3 days. Recently, a new type of automatic positioning system has become available [45]. The improved accuracy of dose planning and shortening of the treatment time are the main advantages of automatic positioning system.

Cumulative cases treated in Japan and worldwide are summarized in Table 1. Metastatic brain tumors are the most common lesion treated by GKS, especially in Japan.

Table 1 Types of Tumor Treated to December 2004

	Japan	Worldwide
Vascular Disorders		
Arteriovenous Malformation	10.9%	13.4%
Aneurysm	0.0%	0.1%
Cavernous Angiomas	0.1%	0.1%
Other Vascular Disorders	0.6%	1.1%
Benign Tumors		
Vestibular Schwannoma	8.2%	9.5%
Trigeminal Schwannoma	0.6%	0.6%
Other Schwannoma	0.5%	0.2%
Benign Glial Tumors (Grade I+II)	0.1%	0.2%
Meningioma	9.0%	12.3%
Pituitary Adenoma (Secreting)	2.3%	5.3%
Pituitary Adenoma (Non-secreting)	1.3%	3.0%
Pineal Region Tumor	0.4%	0.9%
Hemangioblastoma	0.4%	0.4%
Hemangiopericytoma	0.2%	0.3%
Craniopharyngioma	1.0%	0.9%
Chordoma	0.4%	0.4%
Glomus Tumor	0.1%	0.3%
Other Benign Tumors	0.6%	0.8%
Malignant Tumors		
Malignant Glial Tumor (Grade III+IV)	4.9%	6.9%
Metastatic Tumor	56.2%	33.6%
Chondrosarcoma	0.1%	0.1%
Nasopharyngeal Carcinoma	0.4%	0.4%
Other Malignant Tumors	1.9%	1.4%
Functional Disorders		
Trigeminal Neuralgia		6.0%
Parkinson's Disease		0.4%
Intractable Pain		0.2%
Epilepsy		0.6%
Other Functional Disorders		0.2%
Ocular Disorders		
Uveal Melanoma		0.4%
Glaucoma		0.1%

(collected by the Leksell Gamma Knife Society)

Efficacy of GKS for Metastatic Brain Tumors

1. Overall Tumor Growth Control

GKS provides good control of growth for various tumors, such as vestibular schwannoma, pituitary adenoma, meningioma, and malignant tumors. Metastatic brain tumor is the most common type of malignant brain tumor treated by GKS. Metastatic brain tumors account for more than 50% of all treated lesions in Japan as shown in Table 1.

The overall tumor growth control rate at one year has been reported as 77% to 94.8% [7, 29, 35, 49, 53, 54], and the recommended prescribed marginal dose to obtain excellent local control is more than 18 Gy [29, 55]. This high rate of tumor growth control is apparently superior to that of WBRT which achieves tumor growth control of about 50% [61]. The pattern of contrast enhancement is correlated with freedom from progression [55].

Various factors indicate a good prognosis, including age <65 years, higher Karnofsky performance status (KPS), no known extracranial metastases, control of the primary tumor, good recursive partitioning analysis class, smaller tumor volume, interval greater than 2 years between diagnosis of the primary tumor and diagnosis of a single brain metastasis, and lower number of brain metastases [22, 24, 29, 62].

Median survival time was 10 months for patients with metastatic brain tumors treated with direct surgery followed by WBRT, but only 3.75 months for patients treated with only WBRT [41]. Median survival time after GKS has been reported as 7.0-12.3 months [7, 8, 14, 22, 35, 49, 57].

2. GKS for So-called Radioresistant Tumors

GKS can achieve good tumor control even for so-called radioresistant tumors such as renal cell carcinoma and malignant melanoma. GKS has been reported as effective against renal cell carcinoma [36, 42, 47, 52], with more than 90% of tumor growth control. Initial GKS provided an actuarial local control rate of 95% [68], with tumor bleeding in 10% and late radiation toxicity in 20%. The local control rate of 39 treated tumors was 90% and no newly developed neurological deficits were found due to GKS [34]. In a consecutive series of 21 patients, no patients died of progression of intracranial diseases or deteriorated neurological status following GKS [42].

Linac stereotactic radiosurgery or GKS also provides good tumor growth control of cerebral melanoma metastases [14, 25, 32, 33, 48, 71]. The imaging and clinical outcomes of 45 patients with 92 melanoma metastases showed that 24% of treated lesions disappeared, 35% shrank, 23% did not change, and 18% increased in size. Possibly the radiobiological effect of a single high dose overcomes the radioresistant nature of the tumor [32]. Stereotactic radiosurgery controlled 90% of treated melanoma brain metastases for the lifetime of the patients [71].

These results suggest that patients with brain metastases from radioresistant tumors such as renal cell carcinoma and melanoma are especially good candidates for radiosurgery.

However, the survival after stereotactic radiosurgery was significantly worse for patients with melanoma brain metastases compared to patients with renal cell carcinoma [5].

3. GKS for Metastases in the Brain Stem

The tumor location is a very important factor in deciding the treatment strategy, and the brain stem is a difficult location to establish the strategy because of the eloquence and high radiosensitivity. About 0.5-11% of metastatic brain tumors occur in the brain stem [6, 10, 11, 20, 67]. The brain stem is believed to be highly radiosensitive [4, 54], but the evidence for greater sensitivity than the cerebrum is not totally convincing [12]. The marginal dose of stereotactic irradiation for brain stem metastases is recommended to be 15 Gy or less to avoid radiation-induced injury [19]. A marginal dose of 15 Gy or less achieved an overall tumor control rate of 77.4% [58]. Accurate targeting of the tumor and safe dose planning are essential to obtain satisfactory outcomes for patients with brain stem metastases treated by GKS. However, radiosurgery does offer an effective method to treat brain stem metastases.

4. GKS for Metastatic Cystic Tumors

Metastatic cystic brain tumor is not rare and carries an unfavorable prognosis [37]. Large metastatic cystic tumor is not a good candidate for GKS, so cyst aspiration followed by GKS is recommended. Volume reduction by cyst aspiration and insertion of an Ommaya reservoir is possible under local anesthesia. Stereotactic aspiration is also useful for deep-seated cystic tumors [38]. We recommend GKS on the same day or the day after cyst aspiration. However, the viscosity of the cyst content is very high in some cases and effective aspiration is impossible, so GKS combined with external radiation therapy or stereotactic radiotherapy should be considered. Information about the nature of the cyst content is important to obtain before the surgical procedure, but may be difficult in some cases.

5. Complications after Radiosurgery

Complications attributable to local anesthesia or placement of the stereotactic frame are rare, and include fracture of the anterior wall of the frontal sinus and burn at the point of pin fixation. Transient morbidity and mortality rates are 8.9% and 1.8% after GKS [35]. Seizures, nausea, and vomiting are the most common complications. Radiogenic complications such as peritumoral edema usually occur within the first 6 months after radiosurgery [35, 55]. Edema may require the administration of steroids in some symptomatic cases, but is usually transient. The absence of risk of brain atrophy, hair loss, or dementia following GKS is an advantage over WBRT [26].

The presence of pretreatment edema is not correlated with post-radiosurgical complication rates [16]. Therefore, the radiation dose should be adequate for tumors with severe peritumoral edema if the tumor volume is small (less than 2 cm in diameter).

However, a high marginal dose of more than 20 Gy resulted in no better tumor control and greater risk of post-radiosurgical complications [53].

Increased size of the enhanced tumor is not rare after GKS. The differential diagnosis of recurrence of tumor and radiation injury is very important and thallium-201 chloride single photon emission computed tomography or positron emission tomography is useful in many cases [51, 63]. However, the differential diagnosis is sometimes very difficult [21]. If the differential diagnosis is difficult and the mass effect is not negligible, we recommend lesionectomy by direct surgery to obtain the histological diagnosis and stabilize the intracranial pressure.

WBRT and GKS

1. Combination of WBRT and GKS

The advantages of WBRT compared with GKS for the treatment of metastatic tumors remain unclear [2, 27, 28, 60]. GKS plus WBRT may provide better local control or hinder development of new lesions, compared with only GKS [7, 8, 44, 60]. Freedom from progression was worse in patients treated with only radiosurgery compared with radiosurgery plus WBRT initially (28% versus 69%) [62]. However, adjuvant WBRT does not affect survival if successful salvage therapy such as repeated radiosurgery or WBRT was performed [7, 8, 62]. In contrast, GKS plus WBRT achieved better tumor control compared with only WBRT in patients with two to four metastases, as the rate of local failure at 1 year was 100% after only WBRT compared to only 8% after WBRT with boost radiosurgery [27]. There was no difference in overall survival between the two groups.

Study of 1-year survivor with brain metastases treated by stereotactic radiosurgery found that addition of concurrent WBRT to GKS was associated with improved local control rate in subgroups of patients with tumor volume >/=2 cm^3, peripheral dose </=16 Gy, single metastases, nonradioresistant tumors, and specifically lung cancer metastases [66]. Only radiosurgery can achieve high local tumor control rates similar to those achieved by a combination of direct surgery and radiotherapy for patients with single, circumscribed metastases of less than 3.5 cm in diameter [35].

Recently, a randomized trial demonstrated that WBRT and stereotactic boost treatment (including both GKS and Linac-based systems) improves the KPS for all patients and survival for patients with a solitary unresectable lesion [1]. WBRT and stereotactic radiosurgery are recommended for patients with one to three unresectable brain metastases. However, the use of WBRT for patients with one to three brain metastases is still controversial.

Half of the patients initially treated by GKS for metastatic brain tumors did not undergo or require either WBRT or salvage GKS [7]. Therefore, the use of prophylactic WBRT should be carefully considered. On the other hand, radiosurgery with a marginal dose of 20 Gy combined with planned WBRT is recommended as the optimum treatment for metastatic brain tumors of less than 2 cm in diameter [53].

2. Repeated GKS

Repeatability is a major advantage of GKS compared with WBRT. Brain atrophy or dementia following WBRT is also a significant problem [9]. Recently, a multi-institutional review of radiosurgery versus radiosurgery with WBRT as the initial treatment for metastatic brain tumors demonstrated that addition of WBRT to the initial management provided no advantage [62]. There was no difference in survival between the patients who received initial radiosurgery and those who received radiosurgery plus WBRT, even if the Radiation Therapy Oncology Group recursive partitioning analysis class was adjusted [62]. The median survival time is only 37-56 weeks in many patients with metastatic brain tumors [2, 40, 41, 56], so the duration of hospitalization is very important.

We previously reported our experience of repeat GKS for metastatic brain tumors [59]. In this study, the KPS remained relatively good (>70) during the course and only about 30% of patients died of metastatic brain tumors regardless of the presence of multiple newly developed brain metastases. Therefore, we recommend only radiosurgery for metastatic brain tumors or newly developed metastatic lesions after the first GKS rather than WBRT even if fewer than 10-15 multiple tumors are present. Repeat radiosurgery is also reported to be effective [35]. However, the efficacy of multiple repeated GKS is still controversial and a large randomized study is necessary.

3. GKS for Multiple Brain Metastases

WBRT has been used for multiple brain metastases. In addition, GKS has also been used for multiple metastases [49, 50]. The optimum treatment for multiple metastatic brain tumors remains controversial, especially in patients with more than 10 lesions. The number of tumors which can be safely treated and the total dosage delivered to the brain in treating multiple metastatic tumors with GKS should be considered. The upper limit of the daily skull internal dose should be less than 10,000 mJ [49]. Therefore, 20-25 lesions are treatable with GKS if all tumors are less than 1 cm in diameter. Therefore, the maximum number of tumors treatable with GKS may be 25, if the tumors are small and the maximum doses are less than 40 Gy [70]. Treatment of patients with 10 or more metastatic brain tumors by GKS showed that the cumulative WBRT dose was within the threshold level of brain necrosis [69]. A single fraction of GKS is also safe for the treatment of 10 or more simultaneous metastases [65].

New metastases after radiosurgery were found after at least 1-year follow up in 13% of patients with a single metastasis at initial GKS, 34% of patients with two to three metastases, and 100% of patients with four to five metastases [23]. Therefore, only radiosurgery is recommended as the initial treatment for patients with one to three metastases. These findings suggest that further radiosurgery is inevitable in patients with five or more brain metastases if initially treated by only radiosurgery. However, this disadvantage is overcome by the absence of risk of brain atrophy or dementia following GKS. Only radiosurgery is also recommended if the patient has one or two metastases of less than 3 cm in diameter [17]. Despite all these observations, the optimum treatment of multiple metastatic brain tumors remains controversial.

Therapeutic Strategy for Metastatic Brain Tumors

Tumor removal by direct surgery followed by WBRT has been the standard strategy for metastatic brain tumors [41]. GKS may be the first choice for the treatment of metastatic tumors of less than 3 cm in diameter [14, 15]. On the other hand, we recommend direct surgery for tumors of more than 3 cm in diameter, if located in surgically accessible regions. Cyst aspiration under local anesthesia followed by GKS is very useful in some patients with large cystic metastases. We use WBRT for patients with more than 10-15 metastases or cerebrospinal dissemination. Stereotactic radiotherapy (such as cyber knife) or WBRT is recommended for large and surgically unresectable lesions.

References

[1] Andrews DW; Scott CB; Sperduto PW; Flanders AE; Gaspar LE; Schell MC; Werner-Wasik M; Demas W; Ryu J; Bahary JP; Souhami L; Rotman M; Mehta MP; and Curran WJ Jr. (2004). Whole brain radiation therapy with or without stereotactic radiosurgery boost for patients with one to three brain metastases: phase III results of the RTOG 9508 randomised trial. *Lancet*, 363, 1665-1672.

[2] Auchter RM; Lamond JP; Alexander E; Buatti JM; Chappell R; Friedman WA; Kinsella TJ; Levin AB; Noyes WR; Schultz CJ; Loeffler JS; and Mehta MP (1996). A multiinstitutional outcome and prognostic factor analysis of radiosurgery for resectable single brain metastasis. *Int J Radiat Oncol Biol Phys*, 35, 27-35.

[3] Bindal RK; Sawaya R; Leavens ME; and Lee JJ (1993). Surgical treatment of multiple brain metastases. *J Neurosurg*, 79, 210-216.

[4] Boden G (1950). Radiation myelitis of the brain stem. *J Fac Radiol*, 2, 79-94.

[5] Chang EL; Selek U; Hassenbusch SJ 3rd; Maor MH; Allen PK; Mahajan A; Sawaya R; and Woo SY (2005). Outcome variation among "radioresistant" brain metastases treated with stereotactic radiosurgery. *Neurosurgery*, 56, 936-945.

[6] Chason JL; Walker FB; and Landers JW (1963). Metastatic carcinoma in the central nervous system and dorsal root ganglia. A prospective autopsy study. *Cancer*, 16, 781-787.

[7] Chen JC; Petrovich Z; Giannotta SL; Yu C; and Apuzzo ML (2000). Radiosurgical salvage therapy for patients presenting with recurrence of metastatic disease to the brain. *Neurosurgery*, 46, 860-866.

[8] Chidel MA; Suh JH; Reddy CA; Chao ST; Lundbeck MF; and Barnett GH (2000). Application of recursive partitioning analysis and evaluation of the use of whole brain radiation among patients treated with stereotactic radiosurgery for newly diagnosed brain metastases. *Int J Radiat Oncol Biol Phys*, 47, 993-999.

[9] DeAngelis LM; Delattre JY; and Posner JB (1989). Radiation-induced dementia in patients cured of brain metastases. *Neurology*, 39, 789-796.

[10] Delattre JY; Krol G; Thaler HT; and Posner JB (1988). Distribution of brain metastases. *Arch Neurol*, 45, 741-744.

[11] Earle KM (1954). Metastatic and primary intracranial tumors of the adult male. *J Neuropathol Exp Neurol*, 13, 448-454.

[12] Emami B; Lyman J; Brown A; Coia L; Goitein M; Munzenrider JE; Shank B; Solin LJ; and Wesson M (1991). Tolerance of normal tissue to therapeutic irradiation. *Int J Radiat Oncol Biol Phys*, 21, 109-122.

[13] Engenhart R; Kimmig BN; Hover KH; Wowra B; Romahn J; Lorenz WJ; van Kaick G; and Wannenmacher M (1993). Long-term follow-up for brain metastases treated by percutaneous stereotactic single high-dose irradiation. *Cancer*, 71, 1353-1361.

[14] Flickinger JC; Kondziolka D; Lunsford LD; Coffey RJ; Goodman ML; Shaw EG; Hudgins WR; Weiner R; Harsh GR 4th; Sneed PK; and Larson DA (1994). A multi-institutional experience with stereotactic radiosurgery for solitary brain metastasis. *Int J Radiat Oncol Biol Phys*, 28, 797-802.

[15] Flickinger JC; and Kondziolka D (1996). Radiosurgery instead of resection for solitary brain metastasis: The gold standard redefined. *Int J Radiat Oncol Biol Phys*, 35, 185-186.

[16] Gelblum DY; Lee H; Bilsky M; Pinola C; Longford S; and Wallner K (1998). Radiographic findings and morbidity in patients treated with stereotactic radiosurgery. *Int J Radiat Oncol Biol Phys*, 42, 391-395.

[17] Hasegawa T; Kondziolka D; Flickinger JC; Germanwala A; and Lunsford LD (2003). Brain metastases treated with radiosurgery alone: an alternative to whole brain radiotherapy? *Neurosurgery*, 52, 1318-1326.

[18] Hazuka MB; and Kinzie JJ (1988). Brain metastases: results and effects of re-irradiation. *Int J Radiat Oncol Biol Phys*, 15, 433-437.

[19] Huang CF; Kondziolka D; Flickinger JC; and Lunsford LD (1999). Stereotactic radiosurgery for brainstem metastases. *J Neurosurg*, 91, 563-568.

[20] Hunter KMF; and Rewcastle NB (1968). Metastatic neoplasms of the brain stem. *Can Med Assoc J*, 98, 1-7.

[21] Iwai Y; Yamanaka K; Oda J; Tsuyuguchi N; and Ochi H (2001). Tracer accumulation in radiation necrosis of the brain after thallium-201 SPECT and [^{11}C]methionine PET--case report. *Neurol Med Chir* (Tokyo), 41, 415-418.

[22] Jawahar A; Matthew RE; Minagar A; Shukla D; Zhang JH; Willis BK; Ampil F; and Nanda A (2004). Gamma knife surgery in the management of brain metastases from lung carcinoma: a retrospective analysis of survival, local tumor control, and freedom from new brain metastasis. *J Neurosurg*, 100, 842-847.

[23] Kihlstrom L; Karlsson B; and Lindquist C (1993). Gamma Knife surgery for cerebral metastases. Implications for survival based on 16 years experience. *Stereotact Funct Neurosurg*, 61 Suppl 1, 45-50.

[24] Kim DG; Chung HT; Gwak HS; Paek SH; Jung HW; and Han DH (2000). Gamma knife radiosurgery for brain metastases: prognostic factors for survival and local control. *J Neurosurg*, 93 Suppl 3, 23-29.

[25] Koc M; McGregor J; Grecula J; Bauer CJ; Gupta N; and Gahbauer RA (2005). Gamma Knife radiosurgery for intracranial metastatic melanoma: an analysis of survival and prognostic factors. *J Neurooncol*, 71, 307-313.

[26] Kondziolka D; Niranjan A; Flickinger JC; and Lunsford LD (2005). Radiosurgery with or without whole-brain radiotherapy for brain metastases: the patients' perspective regarding complications. *Am J Clin Oncol*, 28, 173-179.

[27] Kondziolka D; Patel A; Lunsford LD; Kassam A; and Flickinger JC (1999). Stereotactic radiosurgery plus whole brain radiotherapy versus radiotherapy alone for patients with multiple brain metastases. *Int J Radiat Oncol Biol Phys*, 45, 427-434.

[28] Li B; Yu J; Suntharalingam M; Kennedy AS; Amin PP; Chen Z; Yin R; Guo S; Han T; Wang Y; Yu N; Song G; and Wang L (2000). Comparison of three treatment options for single brain metastasis from lung cancer. *Int J Cancer*, 90, 37-45.

[29] Lutterbach J; Cyron D; Henne K; and Ostertag CB (2003). Radiosurgery followed by planned observation in patients with one to three brain metastases. *Neurosurgery*, 52, 1066-1073.

[30] Mandell L; Hilaris B; Sullivan M; Sundaresan N; Nori D; Kim JH; Martini N; and Fuks Z (1986). The treatment of single brain metastasis from non-oat cell lung carcinoma. Surgery and radiation versus radiation therapy alone. *Cancer*, 58, 641-649.

[31] Mehta MP; Rozental JM; Levin AB; Mackie TR; Kubsad SS; Gehring MA; and Kinsella TJ (1992). Defining the role of radiosurgery in the management of brain metastases. *Int J Radiat Oncol Biol Phys*, 24, 619-625.

[32] Mingione V; Oliveira M; Prasad D; Steiner M; and Steiner L (2002). Gamma surgery for melanoma metastases in the brain. *J Neurosurg*, 96, 544-551.

[33] Mori Y; Kondziolka D; Flickinger JC; Kirkwood JM; Agarwala S; and Lunsford LD (1998). Stereotactic radiosurgery for cerebral metastatic melanoma: factors affecting local disease control and survival. *Int J Radiat Oncol Biol Phys*, 42, 581-589.

[34] Mori Y; Kondziolka D; Flickinger JC; Logan T; and Lunsford LD (1998). Stereotactic radiosurgery for brain metastasis from renal cell carcinoma. *Cancer*, 83, 344-353.

[35] Muacevic A; Kreth FW; Horstmann GA; Schmid-Elsaesser R; Wowra B; Steiger HJ; and Reulen HJ (1999). Surgery and radiotherapy compared with gamma knife radiosurgery in the treatment of solitary cerebral metastases of small diameter. *J Neurosurg*, 91, 35-43.

[36] Muacevic A; Kreth FW; Mack A; Tonn JC; and Wowra B (2004). Stereotactic radiosurgery without radiation therapy providing high local tumor control of multiple brain metastases from renal cell carcinoma. *Minim Invasive Neurosurg*, 47, 203-208.

[37] Nakagawa H; Kimura S; Kubo S; Fujita T; Tsuruzono K; and Hayakawa T (1992). Prognostic factors in patients surviving for more than 1 or 5 years after removal of metastatic brain tumors. *Neurol Med Chir* (Tokyo), 32, 947-951.

[38] Niranjan A; Witham T; Kondziolka D; and Lunsford LD (2000). The role of stereotactic cyst aspiration for glial and metastatic brain tumors. *Can J Neurol Sci*, 27, 229-235.

[39] Nisce LZ; Hilaris BS; and Chu FC (1971). A review of experience with irradiation of brain metastasis. Am J Roentgenol Radium *Ther Nucl Med*, 111, 329-333.

[40] Noordijk EM; Vecht CJ; Haaxma-Reiche H; Padberg GW; Voormolen JH; Hoekstra FH; Tans JT; Lambooij N; Metsaars JA; Wattendorff AR; Brand R; and Hermans J (1994). The choice of treatment of single brain metastasis should be based on extracranial tumor activity and age. *Int J Radiat Oncol Biol Phys*, 29, 711-717.

[41] Patchell RA; Tibbs PA; Walsh JW; Dempsey RJ; Maruyama Y; Kryscio RJ; Markesbery WR; Macdonald JS; and Young B (1990) A randomized trial of surgery in the treatment of single metastases to the brain. *N Engl J Med*, 322, 494-500.

[42] Payne BR; Prasad D; Szeifert G; Steiner M; and Steiner L (2000). Gamma surgery for intracranial metastases from renal cell carcinoma. *J Neurosurg*, 92, 760-765.

[43] Pickren JW; Lopez G; and Tsukada Y (1983). Brain metastases. An autopsy study. *Cancer Treat Symp*, 2, 295-313.

[44] Pirzkall A; Debus J; Lohr F; Fuss M; Rhein B; Engenhart-Cabillic R; and Wannenmacher M (1998). Radiosurgery alone or in combination with whole-brain radiotherapy for brain metastases. *J Clin Oncol*, 16, 3563-3569.

[45] Regis J; Hayashi M; Porcheron D; Delsanti C; Muracciole X; and Peragut JC (2002). Impact of the model C and Automatic Positioning System on gamma knife radiosurgery: an evaluation in vestibular schwannomas. *J Neurosurg*, 97(5 Suppl), 588-591.

[46] Salerno TA; Munro DD; and Little JR (1978). Surgical treatment of bronchogenic carcinoma with a brain metastasis. *J Neurosurg*, 48, 350-354.

[47] Schoggl A; Kitz K; Ertl A; Dieckmann K; Saringer W; and Koos WT (1998). Gamma-knife radiosurgery for brain metastases of renal cell carcinoma: results in 23 patients. *Acta Neurochir* (Wien), 140, 549-555.

[48] Selek U; Chang EL; Hassenbusch SJ 3rd; Shiu AS; Lang FF; Allen P; Weinberg J; Sawaya R; and Maor MH (2004). Stereotactic radiosurgical treatment in 103 patients for 153 cerebral melanoma metastases. *Int J Radiat Oncol Biol Phys*, 59, 1097-1106.

[49] Serizawa T; Iuchi T; Ono J; Saeki N; Osato K; Odaki M; Ushikubo O; Hirai S; Sato M; and Matsuda S (2000). Gamma knife treatment for multiple metastatic brain tumors compared with whole-brain radiation therapy. *J Neurosurg*, 93 Suppl 3, 32-36.

[50] Serizawa T; Saeki N; Higuchi Y; Ono J; Iuchi T; Nagano O; and Yamaura A (2005). Gamma knife surgery for brain metastases: indications for and limitations of a local treatment protocol. *Acta Neurochir* (Wien), 147, 721-726.

[51] Serizawa T; Saeki N; Higuchi Y; Ono J; Matsuda S; Sato M; Yanagisawa M; Iuchi T; Nagano O; and Yamaura A (2005). Diagnostic value of thallium-201 chloride single-photon emission computerized tomography in differentiating tumor recurrence from radiation injury after gamma knife surgery for metastatic brain tumors. *J Neurosurg*, 102 Suppl, 266-271.

[52] Sheehan JP; Sun MH; Kondziolka D; Flickinger J; and Lunsford LD (2003). Radiosurgery in patients with renal cell carcinoma metastasis to the brain: long-term outcomes and prognostic factors influencing survival and local tumor control. *J Neurosurg*, 98, 342-349.

[53] Shehata MK; Young B; Reid B; Patchell RA; St Clair W; Sims J; Sanders M; Meigooni A; Mohiuddin M; and Regine WF (2004). Stereotactic radiosurgery of 468 brain

metastases < or =2 cm: implications for SRS dose and whole brain radiation therapy. *Int J Radiat Oncol Biol Phys*, 59, 87-93.

[54] Sheline GE; Wara WM; and Smith V (1980). Therapeutic irradiation and brain injury. *Int J Radiat Oncol Biol Phys*, 6, 1215-1228.

[55] Shiau CY; Sneed PK; Shu HK; Lamborn KR; McDermott MW; Chang S; Nowak P; Petti PL; Smith V; Verhey LJ; Ho M; Park E; Wara WM; Gutin PH; and Larson DA (1997). Radiosurgery for brain metastases: relationship of dose and pattern of enhancement to local control. *Int J Radiat Oncol Biol Phys*, 37, 375-383.

[56] Shirato H; Takamura A; Tomita M; Suzuki K; Nishioka T; Isu T; Kato T; Sawamura Y; Miyamachi K; Abe H; and Miyasaka K (1997). Stereotactic irradiation without whole-brain irradiation for single brain metastasis. *Int J Radiat Oncol Biol Phys*, 37, 385-391.

[57] Shu HKG; Sneed PK; Shiau CY; McDermott MW; Lamborn KR; Park E; Ho M; Petti PL; Smith V; Verhey LJ; Wara WM; Gutin PH; and Karson DA (1996). Factors influencing survival after gamma knife radiosurgery for patients with single and multiple brain metastases. *Cancer J Sci Am*, 2, 335-342.

[58] Shuto T; Fujino H; Asada H; Inomori S; and Nagano H (2003). Gamma knife radiosurgery for metastatic tumours in the brain stem. *Acta Neurochir* (Wien), 145, 755-760.

[59] Shuto T; Fujino H; Inomori S; and Nagano H (2004). Repeated gamma knife radiosurgery for multiple metastatic brain tumours. *Acta Neurochir* (Wien), 146, 989-993.

[60] Sneed PK; Lamborn KR; Forstner JM; McDermott MW; Chang S; Park E; Gutin PH; Phillips TL; Wara WM; and Larson DA (1999). Radiosurgery for brain metastases: is whole brain radiotherapy necessary? *Int J Radiat Oncol Biol Phys*, 43, 549-558.

[61] Sneed PK; Larson DA; and Wara WM (1996). Radiotherapy for cerebral metastases. *Neurosurg Clin N Am*, 7, 505-515.

[62] Sneed PK; Suh JH; Goetsch SJ; Sanghavi SN; Chappell R; Buatti JM; Regine WF; Weltman E; King VJ; Breneman JC; Sperduto PW; and Mehta MP (2002). A multi-institutional review of radiosurgery alone vs. radiosurgery with whole brain radiotherapy as the initial management of brain metastases. *Int J Radiat Oncol Biol Phys*, 53, 519-526.

[63] Sonoda Y; Kumabe T; Takahashi T; Shirane R; and Yoshimoto T (1998). Clinical usefulness of ^{11}C-MET PET and ^{201}Tl SPECT for differentiation of recurrent glioma from radiation necrosis. *Neurol Med Chir* (Tokyo), 38, 342-347.

[64] Sturm V; Kober B; Hover KH; Schlegel W; Boesecke R; Pastyr O; Hartmann GH; Schabbert S; zum Winkel K; Kunze S; and Lorenz WJ (1987). Stereotactic percutaneous single dose irradiation of brain metastases with a linear accelerator. *Int J Radiat Oncol Biol Phys*, 13, 279-282.

[65] Suzuki S; Omagari J; Nishio S; Nishiye E; and Fukui M (2000). Gamma knife radiosurgery for simultaneous multiple metastatic brain tumors. *J Neurosurg*, 93 Suppl 3, 30-31.

[66] Varlotto JM; Flickinger JC; Niranjan A; Bhatnagar A; Kondziolka D; and Lunsford LD (2005). The impact of whole-brain radiation therapy on the long-term control and

morbidity of patients surviving more than one year after gamma knife radiosurgery for brain metastases. *Int J Radiat Oncol Biol Phys*, 62, 1125-1132.

[67] White KT; Fleming TR; and Laws ER Jr (1981). Single metastasis to the brain. Surgical treatment in 122 consecutive patients. *Mayo Clin Proc*, 56, 424-428.

[68] Wowra B; Siebels M; Muacevic A; Kreth FW; Mack A; and Hofstetter A (2002). Repeated gamma knife surgery for multiple brain metastases from renal cell carcinoma. *J Neurosurg*, 97, 785-793.

[69] Yamamoto M; Ide M; Nishio S; and Urakawa Y (2002). Gamma knife radiosurgery for numerous brain metastases: Is this a safe treatment? *Int J Radiat Oncol Biol Phys*, 53, 1279-1283.

[70] Yang CC; Ting J; Wu X; and Markoe A (1998). Dose volume histogram analysis of the gamma knife radiosurgery treating twenty-five metastatic intracranial tumors. *Stereotact Funct Neurosurg*, 70 Suppl 1, 41-49.

[71] Yu C; Chen JC; Apuzzo ML; O'Day S; Giannotta SL; Weber JS; and Petrovich Z (2002). Metastatic melanoma to the brain: prognostic factors after gamma knife radiosurgery. *Int J Radiat Oncol Biol Phys*, 52, 1277-1287.

[72] Yuh WT; Tali ET; Nguyen HD; Simonson TM; Mayr NA; and Fisher DJ (1995). The effect of contrast dose, imaging time, and lesion size in the MR detection of intracerebral metastasis. *AJNR Am J Neuroradiol*, 16, 373-380.

In: Brain Cancer Therapy and Surgical Interventions... ISBN 1-59454-974-5
Editor: Andrew V. Yang, pp. 127-145

Chapter VI

Advances in the Radiotherapy of Pediatric Brain Tumors

Marzanna Chojnacka [*] ***and Anna Skowrońska-Gardas***
The Maria Skłodowska-Curie Memorial Cancer Center and Institute, Warsaw, Poland

Abstract

Primary central nervous system neoplasm's (CNS) are the most frequent solid tumors in childhood. Despite developments in neurosurgery, radiotherapy and chemotherapy, a significant proportion of these patients suffer progressive disease. A good treatment management strategy should consider not only survival but also the quality of life of the child. Irradiation is an essential part in the management of the majority of CNS tumors. During the last decade, there were significant advances in the technology of planning and delivery of radiation treatment.

Conformal radiotherapy techniques are performed using multiple treatment fields; each shaped to conform to the beam's eye view of the target volume. It allows a high homogenous dose to the tumor region with minimizing doses to normal tissue. This is particularly important for children with localized low-grade tumors, whose prognosis of long- term survival is often excellent and should be accompanied by smallest possible risk of the treatment toxicity.

Many reports stress the impact of radiotherapy technical quality on survival. In our report the protracted irradiation and correctness of whole brain fields may be a major contributing factor for the overall outcome in children with medulloblastoma.

The new approach of radiotherapy such a conformal, intensity modulated photon beam and stereotactic methods have recently been developed. These new methods in therapy of pediatric brain tumors and our experience in treatment of children with

---

[*] Correspondence to: Marzanna Chojnacka, 1st Department of Radiotherapy, The Maria Skłodowska-Curie Memorial Cancer Center and Institute, 00-973 Warsaw, Wawelska 15, Poland, e-mail: marzanna.ch1@wp.pl

medulloblastoma, low-grade astrocytoma, craniopharyngioma and brain stem tumors are presented.

We summarized therapeutic aspects of most childhood brain tumors.

Introduction

Tumors of the central nervous system (CNS) are the most common form of solid tumors in childhood, accounting for 20% of all pediatric malignancies. Half of all pediatric brain tumors are located within the posterior fossa, and with the exception of cerebellar astrocytoma, most of these tumors require radiation therapy [1].

Currently radiation therapy is going trough a dynamic period. New imaging tools (spiral CT, MRI, PET, CT-PET etc.) enable more accurate outlining of the target volumes and organs at risk. Advanced techniques for radiation therapy treatment planning and delivery have been implemented for clinical use with the aim of reducing radiation-related side effects and safely increasing the dose of radiation delivered to the volume considered at risk. For most childhood tumors, dose escalation has not been a priority. Toxicity reduction is a principal goal, with a potential to reduce late effects of therapy and make radiotherapy safer for children of all ages [2, 3].

In conformal therapy the idea is to create irregularly shaped fields adjusted to the clinical target volume (CTV) with margins from each beam direction. Each beam is conformed to the projection of the planning target volume (PTV) either by a conformal lead alloy block or a multileaf collimator (MLC) using tree-dimensional reconstruction and beam's eye view facilities. The goal is then usually to cover the CTV with a homogenous dose and to avoid risk organs [2, 4-7].

Intensity-modulated radiation therapy (IMRT) is capable of generating complex tree-dimensional dose distribution to conform closely to the target volume. With IMRT, the beam intensity is optimized, using computer algorithms, as it is oriented around the patient. This process is based on the "inverse method" of treatment planning and is capable of generating significant dose gradients between the target volume and adjacent tissue structures to accomplish the intended dose-volume prescription [6, 8].

The aim of stereotactically guided conformal radiotherapy (SCRT) is a high-precision technique for the delivery of highly conformal dose distribution to the target volume using conventional fractionation schemes. By accurate immobilization and treatment delivery, planning target volume (PTV) could involve smaller margins associated with patient movement and setup errors, than for other techniques using conventional immobilization devices [6, 9, 10]. The most frequent patient eligibility criteria for SCRT includes the following histologic subtypes: subtotally resected or progressive craniopharyngioma ≤ 5cm in the maximal dimension, symptomatic or progressive low-grade astrocytoma ≤ 5cm, and well-differentiated ependymoma ≤ 5cm after complete resection [11]. Reducing the irradiated volume is in important goal in the treatment of pediatric CNS tumors. The use of smaller CTV in the posterior fossa tumors resulted in significant sparing of cochleae, pituitary-hypothalamic axis and remaining brain [12-14].

Stereotactic radiosurgery (SRS) utilizes precise head immobilization, CT or MRI imaging, and multiple intersecting beams to deliver a large single fraction of radiation to a small CTV, with significant sparing of surrounding normal tissue. In cases in which residual or recurrent tumor is focally unresectable, an SRS boost should be considered, because it can provide durable local control [15].

Proton beam radiation for malignant tumors may offer clinical advantages for patients with some types of neoplasms. Proton radiotherapy can allow high doses of radiation to be delivered near critical structures, the result of its Bragg peak effect and its finite range. The basis for the advantages is a better dose distribution of the proton radiation. This means that smaller volumes of normal tissues are irradiated, reducing the risk of adverse events, because the adverse events from radiotherapy are both dose-dependent and volume-dependent [6, 16, 17].

Low-grade Astrocytoma

Low-grade astrocytomas (LGG) account for one-third to one-half of all CNS tumors in children. They are a heterogeneous group of tumors with overall survival as high as 80%-100% [1, 7, 10, 11, 18].

The treatment is controversial and is influenced by tumor location and resectability.

Resection remains the preferred treatment for patients with cerebellar and cerebral hemispheric tumors and frequently is curative if a macroscopic total or nearly total resection is achieved. However, for patients with midline and other tumors for whom extensive resection is not possible, the most appropriate management remains undefined.

Local radiotherapy is an effective treatment modality for inoperable and progressive LGGs of childhood, with long-term tumor control rates of 80-90% and 10-year survival rates ranging from 63% to 89% [7, 10, 11]. Late effects in the form of endocrine dysfunction, neurocognitive deficits, and second malignant neoplasms have been attributed to radiotherapy. For this reason, chemotherapy is the first-line treatment for very young children, with the aim of delaying definitive irradiation [19]. The recognition and importance of radiation-induced sequelae have stimulated investigation of alternative treatment approaches, especially the introduction of modern treatment techniques which have the potential to limit the high-dose regions to the tumor itself, thereby reducing the dose to surrounding normal tissue. Today, low-grade glioma are therefore a challenging issue for the radiooncologist, because the use of modern technologies would ideally lead to a decrease in long-term toxicity while maintaining or even improving the overall outcome [2, 7, 10, 11].

Stereotactic radiotherapy (SRT) uses highly focal, precise, fractionated irradiation. This method combines the advantages of focused precision radiotherapy with the biologic advantages of fractionation. The precise technical details, as well as the required safety margins, have not been agreed on. The current european recommendation for conventional radiotherapy is a safety margin of 0,5-1cm around pilocytic and 1-2 cm around the GTV of other LGGs. The precision of SRT may allow an additional reduction in the GTV-PTV margins. These margins used by many centers were 7mm and for radiosurgery 2-3 mm [7, 10, 11, 15].

Marcus et al. prospectively studied the efficacy and toxicity of SRT in children with small, localized low-grade brain tumors. The PFS and OS rate was 82,5% and 97,8%, respectively, at 5 years. No recurrences developed at the margin, supporting the use of limited margins. Treatment was well tolerated [11].

Between 1994 and 1999, 14 children with LGGs were treated with fractionated SRT at the Royal Marsden Hospital. The 3-years local PFS and OS rate was 87% and 100%, respectively, compared with 89% and 98% for an historic control treated with conventional radiotherapy. Four of 12 children with neurological deficits improved and 5 remained stable [10].

In our Radiotherapy Department, in 1997-2001, 12 children with LGG were treated with conformal techniques. These patients were treated after partial resection (3) or biopsy (9) and chemotherapy as well (7). Radiotherapy was delivered with linear accelerator with energy 6 or 15 MeV to a total dose 54 Gy in 30 fractions for all patients. Median follow-up was 48 months. Four patients died; three due to tumor progression after 6, 9 and 12 months; one due to complications after chemotherapy. Two children are living with metastases to supratentorial and spinal regions, diagnosed 6 and 16 months post radiotherapy. Four children are living with no evidence of disease and two with MRI proven stable disease. Late complications of radiotherapy were not observed, but longer follow-up is necessary [20].

Conformal radiotherapy is treatment of choice for patients with LGG, when total resection of tumor is not possible. The risk of radiation related complications are relatively low [2, 7, 11, 20].

Malignant Gliomas

Malignant gliomas represent approximately 6% of brain tumors in children. Children have an increased proportion of anaplastic astrocytomas among the malignant gliomas and have longer survival than adults [1].

Surgical resection has often been limited in extent to the poorly circumscribed nature of the tumor. A gross total resection is possible in approximately 25% in cerebral malignant glioma in this age group. There seems to be a significant correlation between degree of resection (especially gross total vs. incomplete removal) and survival; with survival rates after gross total resections exceed 60% at 3 years [21].

Radiation therapy is a primary component of initial management of pediatric malignant gliomas. Adult studies have documented the impact of adequate radiation therapy on survival. The treatment volume should include the macroscopic preoperative tumor and 2 cm safety margin [22]. A dose response suggesting treatment is to at least the 55-60 Gy with conventional fractionation. No clear benefit with hyperfractionation with doses above 70 Gy or accelerated fractionation was obtained [23].

Due to poor results, especially among patients with residual tumor after surgery (the progression - free survival - rate 15-20%), considerable attention has been focused on examining the efficacy of various chemotherapeutic strategies for enhancing disease control. A variety of single agents and combined chemotherapy regimes are under investigation. All of these regiments have demonstrated efficacy in producing objective responses, although their ability to improve disease control over that achieved with standard treatment remains problematic [24].

Brain Stem Tumors

Tumors arising in the midbrain, pons, and medulla oblongata account for 10 to 20% of all central nervous system tumors in the pediatric age group. Their location was thought to preclude surgery as a therapeutic option and patients were usually treated without histologic confirmation of diagnosis with radiotherapy alone. Results of treatment were worse than for any other CNS tumor with 5-year survival rates commonly in the 20 to 30% range [1, 25, 26].

These tumors are grouped as focal, dorsal exophytic, cervicomedullary and diffuse intrinsic tumors. Surgery is the treatment of choice for focal tumors at other locations that are surgically accessible and have imaging characteristics suggestive of low-grade histology. For completely resected low grade astrocytoma results are excellent with freedom from progression in as many as 94% or even 100% of cases [25].

Diffuse intrinsic tumors account for approximately 80% of all brain stem tumors. Majority of them is fibrillary astrocytoma. Neuraxis dissemination is not rare, it occurred within 1 month of local progression in nearly 30% of patients. Surgery has no role in the management of patients with these tumors. The biopsy is no longer considered necessary because in the context of a typical clinical symptoms and MRI findings. For these nonoperable lesions, standard treatment should be considered to be external beam radiotherapy, using limited treatment volumes with margins 1-2 cm, to total dose 54 Gy, given in once daily fractions, over 6 weeks. Stereotactic fractionated radiotherapy, but not radiosurgery, could be an option. Treated with conventional radiotherapy, 80% of patients will improve clinically, but overall survival rates at 2 years are less than 20% [3, 25-27].

Over the past decade, the hyperfractionated radiotherapy (HRT) with higher total dose of radiotherapy was applied in many clinical trials. The tolerance of treatment was good and the early results are encouraging, but it was not confirmed in longer follow-up [23, 28-30]. In 1992, phase III prospective randomized trial POG 9239 was begun comparing hyperfractionated to conventional radiotherapy, with cisplatin used in both study arms. For the patients treated with hyperfractionated regime, 2-years survival was 6,7% and with conventional regime 7,1%. The major conclusion from this trial is that the hyperfractionated method of radiotherapy did not improve event-free survival nor did not improve survival over the conventional regimen, and both treatment are associated with the poor disease - free and survival outcome [31].

The role of conventional chemotherapy as well as high dose chemotherapy has been investigated. Unfortunately, survival using the aggressive treatment modality does not appear to be any better than that reported for conventional radiotherapy [32-33]. Moreover, a detrimental effect of combined chemotherapy - radiotherapy approach in children treated with hyperfractionated radiotherapy plus cisplatinum on POG 9239 was observed, because that survival for these patients was worse than that for patients receiving the same radiotherapy alone on POG 8495. This finding should serve as a caution to those planning aggressive treatment programs in patients with this disease [30].

There are a few publications about the late effects of radiotherapy and quality of life in pediatric brain tumor survivors. We evaluated the quality of life in 19 children with brain stem tumor treated with radiotherapy. From 1982 till 1995, 95 children with this diagnosis were irradiated in our Radiotherapy Department. Radiotherapy for all patients was delivered with a Co60 unit. The treatment volume consisted of the tumor site established on CT or MRI scans, with 2-cm margin. Opposed lateral fields were used. Two regimens of fractionation were applied: conventionally to a total dose of 54 Gy and hyperfractionated: 62,1 Gy in 1,15 Gy twice a day. After mean follow-up 146,5 months, there are 19 of long-term survivors, 10/71 (14%) with diffuse intrinsic tumors and 9/24 (37,5%) with more localized types. Three patients have no symptoms of their disease, and no treatment related complications. Fourteen patients suffered from neurological deficits, but all of them were diagnosed before radiotherapy. Eight patients suffered from hearing loss, ten from endocrine abnormalities. Nine patients reported school difficulties, but they are mild. These complications were observed in a similar proportion in children treated with conventional and hyperfractionated radiotherapy [34].

In conclusion, the prognosis for children with brain stem tumors treated with radiotherapy remains poor, independent of the type of fractionation and total dose applied, but there is a proportion of patients who are long- term survivors. They suffer predominantly from pre-treatment neurological impairment, which seriously influence their quality of life. The most often observed treatment related sequelae such a pituitary insufficiency and hearing loss may be diminished with the application of modern techniques as 3D conformal and intensity modulated radiotherapy.

Medulloblastoma

Medulloblastoma is a highly malignant, infratentorial, neuroectodermal tumor accounting for 20% of all pediatric brain tumors. This is the classic CNS tumor associated with cerebrospinal fluid seeding and metastases. Subarachnoid dissemination is reported at diagnosis in 10-30% of children [1].

Current therapy for this disease includes maximum surgical resection followed by whole neuraxis radiation plus a boost to the posterior fossa, and chemotherapy. Despite this aggressive treatment, only 60% of children with medulloblastoma will be cured, and most of these will suffer long-term side effects [35-37]. At present, children with medulloblastoma are divided into two disease risk groups: average-risk (AR) patients are those diagnosed when they are older than the age of 3 years with nonmetastatic and totally or near-totally resected (≤1,5cm on postoperative MRI scan) disease; patients not fulfilling these criteria are regarded as high-risk (HR) [38-40].

There is considerable data indicating a correlation between dose to the posterior fossa primary site and outcome. Local disease control and survival have been related to posterior fossa doses 50-55 Gy. The proper neuraxis radiation dose to the full brain and spinal canal is more difficult to define. There are number of clinical trials investigating reduced doses for CNS with neoadjuvant and adjuvant chemotherapy for patients with minimal risk of relapse. Early results are encouraging, but longer follow up is necessary. Standard doses for whole

CNS are 35-36 Gy for HR, and 23-25 Gy for AR patients, given in 4 weeks, one a day schedule, followed by boost to posterior fossa to 55 Gy [38, 41]. The prolongation of treatment duration could significantly effect the outcome in terms of control of disease in the posterior fossa and freedom from relapse [42, 43].

The planning and delivery of craniospinal irradiation (CSI) have to be of the highest quality. This is one of the most complex radiotherapy techniques employed in most oncology departments. The accuracy of this contributes to the probability of long-term survival [43-47]. In classical treatment planning there are many problems, such as the junction of craniospinal fields, determination of the inferior border of the thecal sac, patterns of local failure, especially in the cribriform plate and the temporal fossa or the range of posterior fossa boost volume [14, 39, 43-45, 48-51].

The majority of centers use techniques that utilize large lateral whole-brain fields, whose lower borders are carefully matched to the upper border of one or more spinal fields. Blocks are used to shield the lenses, nasal and oral structures. It is essential to avoid shielding meninges, cribriform plate, temporal fossa and base of skull. Because of the close proximity of the lens and the cribriform plate it may be impossible to irradiate the cribriform region adequately and shield the lenses. In irradiated medulloblastoma patients, 10-30% of all failures occurs in the supratentorial region. The majority of these failures were found in the inferior part of frontal and temporal regions. Several authors as a reason for recurrence in this region have mentioned insufficient coverage of the cribriform plate [39, 43, 46, 47, 50, 52]. Miralbell et al. reported an association between supratentorial failure-free survival and field correctness. At 75% patients of all who failed in the supratentorial region, underdosage to the inferior parts of the brain was observed [47]. With current cataract surgical techniques, shielding of the lens is a secondary objective.

The lower border of the spinal field is generally placed at the lower border of the second sacral vertebra. It is important to individualize this because the lower border of the thecal sac can be as high as L5 or as low as S3. This border should be based on MRI [39, 49].

The paradigm of delivering high-dose radiation therapy to the entire posterior fossa for medulloblastoma has been challenged. It is possible to consider tree-dimensional conformal planning to reduce the radiation dose to non-target structures such as the hypothalamus, pituitary gland and middle ear. Minimization of dose to surrounding organs is important in children where various critical structures may not be fully developed [13, 14, 17, 39, 51] . Miralbell have reported no correlation between treatment of the entire posterior cavity and progression-free survival [47]. Some investigators have hypothesized that a high-dose boost to the entire posterior fossa may not be necessary and that a conformal boost limited to the tumor bed plus a margin may be adequate [45, 47, 53].

Children who survive suffer a loss of normal-appearing white matter, an associated decline in intellectual function, and long-term endocrine deficiencies. These adverse effects, which are particularly severe in young patients, are largely the result of neuraxis radiation therapy [39]. Adjuvant chemotherapy allows standard neuraxis radiation for medulloblastoma to be reduced from 36 Gy to 23,4 Gy without affecting cure rates [38]. However, a dose 23,4 Gy is still associated with significant neurotoxicity [37]. COG is planning phase III trial in which children between the ages of 3 and 8 years with newly diagnosed AR medulloblastoma will be randomly assigned to receive either 18 Gy or 23,4 Gy of neuraxis radiation. These additional reductions in radiation treatment may decrease morbidity among surviving patients; however, it remains unclear whether this will occur at the expense of disease control.

In the period from 1983 to 1997, 158 children with medulloblastoma were treated with CSI at the Radiotherapy Department. Children were treated in the prone position with the use of an individually shaped cast for the head. The craniospinal axis was treated at first, followed by a boost to the tumor bed. The cranium was treated with two laterals, opposed fields encompassing the whole brain. The spine was irradiated with a single posterior field or a pair of two abutting fields including the dural sac from C4 to S2 was used. The gaps between fields were planned individually and all the fields' junctions were changed once during the treatment. The median dose prescribed to the CNS was 35 Gy. The primary tumor was boosted to the total dose 55,1 Gy

The technique of radiotherapy was carefully evaluated. Simulation films of the whole brain irradiation fields were retrospectively reviewed. The field margin distances to the cribriform plate and to the floor of the temporal fossa were assessed.

The median follow-up was 74 months (range: 29-187 months). Median survival and the median time to relapse was 49 ± 12 months and 25 ± 5 months, respectively. Five-year overall survival and 5-year disease free survival was 46% and 40%, respectively

We had evaluated the primary sites of failures. Isolated failures were found in posterior fossa, supratentorial region and spine at the same frequency (21%, 24%, 22,5% respectively). The supratentorial irradiation technique was considered insufficient in 43% patients. In all cases of the failure in the cribriform plate, this region was shielded. The field incorrectness was retained as being significantly correlated with isolated supratentorial failure (p=0,049) [43].

Currently in our department the cribriform plate is visualized on the CT images and included in clinical target volume without any margin. In the most patients the adequate lateral fields are used. In few cases, when cribriform plate was outside the 90% isodose, it was irradiated by the additional, anterior, small electron field. This technique is comparable to that, used by Jereb, who tried to improve overall survival by eliminating supratentorial failures with a 15 Gy electron boost to the cribriform plate [52].

In summary, a correlation between technical factors (correctness of whole brain field) and supratentorial failure was confirmed in our study. Protracted radiotherapy has also a negative impact on outcome. It seems that high quality of radiotherapy may be a major contributing factor for the overall outcome. Our findings confirm the necessity of strict radiotherapy quality control procedures.

Ependymoma

Ependymomas are rare neoplasms that constitute about 10% of all primary brain tumors in childhood, and approximately 70% are located in the posterior fossa. Ependymoma can also occur in the spinal cord accounting for 25% of all tumors in this localization. These tumors arise from the ependymal cells lining the ventricular system and the central spinal canal. They have the ability to seed trough the cerebrospinal fluid pathways [1]. The incidence of neuraxis dissemination reported in the literature is approximately 10% for low-grade ependymoma, but 40% for anaplastic tumor [54-56].

The management of intracranial ependymoma is a controversial topic in pediatric neuro-oncology and may range among institutions from surgery alone to a combination of surgery, radiotherapy and chemotherapy. Some of the many questions still under debate concern the optimal radiotherapy volumes, doses and techniques; the use of chemotherapy; and the prognostic impact of histologic grading, patient's age and tumor site.

The 5-year survival for children with ependymoma ranges between 30 and 70%, with a worse prognosis for patients with residual disease after surgery, anaplastic histology and infratentorial localization [54-59].

Radiotherapy is generally accepted as part of the standard treatment for ependymomas, but optimal irradiation modalities are not well defined. Recommendations regarding treatment volume have evolved over the years. In the past these patients were often treated with craniospinal irradiation [60]. However numerous reports have established the efficacy of local fields in management of this tumor [1, 57, 61-65]. The rate of isolated out-of-field failures in patient irradiated with volumes less than craniospinal ranges 0-12,5% [62, 65-67]. Because CSI is associated with considerable late toxicity, especially in children, this pattern of failure does not warrant its routine use. In the current era, with the low risk of neuraxis dissemination at presentation and the knowledge that failure is predominantly local, CSI has been assumed to be unnecessary. Patients with M0 disease should receive local irradiation. For disseminated ependymomas, most radiation oncologists employ craniospinal radiotherapy [3, 66]. What is the local radiotherapy: only tumor bed or the entire posterior fossa? In the retrospective study of infratentorial ependymoma, 9 patients had tumor bed irradiation alone, and 6 did not have radiotherapy. Three patients recurred, and all were in the tumor bed. There were no nontumor bed posterior fossa failures in this subset of children. All had a low-grade tumor [67]. Based on this observation, it seems that the entire posterior fossa need not be treated in nondisseminated low-grade infratentorial ependymomas. Whether the entire posterior fossa should be treated in high-grade infratentorial ependymoma is not known. Based on two retrospective studies of high-grade ependymoma, in which the most common site of failure was local, one can argue to use tumor bed radiotherapy for all M0 patients [56, 68]. Subsequently, the histologic grade has not played a role in the selection of treatment [59]. Currently, radiotherapy is delivered to the tumor bed with a 2-cm safety margin in the high grade, and 1cm- in the low-grade M0 tumors. This information can be used to minimize late effects of irradiation in the era of three-dimensional (conformal) radiotherapy.

Standard radiation therapy doses have been in the area of 50 Gy. Many authors not found relationship between radiation dose and local control for childhood ependymoma [62, 65]. Hyperfractionated radiotherapy, despite the high dose (70,4 Gy), did not change the prognosis of these tumors as compared to conventional fractionation [58]. Currently, most protocols recommend 54 Gy in 30 fractions over 6 weeks for low-grade ependymoma and 59,4 Gy in 33 fractions over 6,5 weeks in high-grade tumor. This scheme represents balance between treatment efficacy and late toxicity. In the last Children's Oncology Group trial for intracranial ependymoma (ACNS 0121) patients with gross total resection of supratentorial grade II tumors will be observed. Other patients with near total or gross total resection will receive conformal radiotherapy to 59,4 Gy. Patients with subtotal resection will receive systemic chemotherapy with possible second-look surgery, depending on chemotherapy response, followed by conformal irradiation to 59,4 Gy.

The specter of radiation-related side effects has motivated investigators to test strategies to delay or avoid the use of radiation in young children. Cooperative group trial testing the use of chemotherapy to delay radiotherapy reported results inferior to those achieved for patients treated with immediate postoperative radiotherapy. Data from Merchant et al. show that pre-RT chemotherapy negatively influenced PFS and OS. These effect was more pronounced among children with progression while receiving chemotherapy. A delay in the administration of irradiation or chemotherapy-induced radioinsensivity has possibly clinical and biologic explanations [59]. Most published reports have found no benefit of routine chemotherapy [60, 69, 70].

The successful application of conformal irradiation to ependymoma in children may improve outcomes by reducing side effects and thereby permit the reintroduction of radiotherapy as a treatment option for very young children. Merchant et al. evaluated neurocognitive function of 88 pediatric patients with ependymoma before and after conformal therapy. Mean scores on all neurocognitive outcomes were within normal limits. This study is unique because it includes children younger than 3 years. Patients in this age group in earlier studies had a worse prognosis than older patients, possibly because of more aggressive tumor biology, reluctance to give postoperative radiotherapy or use of lower doses of irradiation. The results of this study demonstrated a 3-year PFS estimate of 74,7%. The improved rate of disease control may be attributable to factors that include the high proportion patients after gross resection (85%), targeting with tree-dimensional imaging and the relatively high total dose (59,4 Gy). Limited-volume irradiation achieves high rates of disease control and results in stable neurocognitive outcomes [71].

Intracranial Germ Cell Tumors

Intracranial germ cell tumors (GCT) represent 3-11% of pediatric brain neoplasms. Approximately 50% to 65% of these are germinomas. The remainder comprise a heterogenous group of tumors termed nongerminomatous germ cell tumors (NGGCT) which include pure or mixed populations of primitive germ cell elements including embryonal carcinoma, endodermal sinus tumor, choriocarcinoma or teratoma. Typically GCTs are found in midline sites, particularly the pineal and suprasellar regions of the brain [1, 72]. The relationship between histopathology and patient outcome has been well described. Published reports corroborate poorer prognosis for patients with NGGCT compared with those with germinoma [73, 74]. There has been an attempt to reduce the toxicity of treatment in the last decade. These attempts have varied from reducing the dose of radiation, and using chemotherapy alone or in combination with reduced dose radiation to reducing the volume of normal tissue irradiated by stereotactic radiotherapy.

Germinoma represents the most common and prognosticaly favorable subgroup, highly radiosensitive, with a predilection for spread along the ventricles and cerebrospinal fluid pathway. Using radiotherapy alone for these tumors overall survivals of 70-97% at 5-years have been reported [75-77]. Several studies have reported excellent outcome with preirradiation chemotherapy followed by focal radiotherapy [78-80]. A point of controversy has been the appropriate field and dose of radiation. They varied according to the tumor extend, patient age, spinal findings and HCG values [76]. Previous prospective data suggesting the effectiveness of craniospinal irradiation in preventing locoregional recurrence [75, 77]. However, the morbidity of radiotherapy in children, has prompted many investigators to explore approaches that reduce the volume and dose of irradiation. The spinal failure rates <10% in the absence of CSI reported in most studies, do not justify routine incorporation of CSI into treatment strategies for localized germinoma [76, 81-83]. The Societé Française d'Oncologie Pediatrique (SFOP) initiated a multicentre study to replace prophylactic CSI with systemic chemotherapy and to restrict radiotherapy to a focal boost of 40 Gy to the initial tumor volume [78]. Several authors have recommended partial brain fields, for instance, tumor with 2-4 cm margins [82, 83]. However most studies report higher recurrence rates associated with radiation targeting the tumor volume only [78, 80, 81]. In Ogawa study 3 (50%) of 6 patients treated with localized-field experienced relapse partly because of the difficulty in accurately determining the initial GTV before surgery and chemotherapy [76]. Haas-Kogan reviewed the irradiation fields of 21 patients with germinoma. No recurrence took place after whole-ventricular fields, 1 intracranial relapse occurred among 3 patients treated to the initial tumor volume, although this patient received only 11 Gy [73]. In this respect most authors recommended whole-ventricular or larger field irradiation followed by a primary tumor boost as a standard treatment for most cases of nonmetastatic intracranial germinoma [73, 79, 80, 84, 85]. For patients with positive tumor cells in the cerebrospinal fluid or tumor deposits by MRI, craniospinal radiotherapy is still recommended as standard therapy [85]. A total dose of 40-50 Gy to adequate treatment fields is effective in preventing intracranial relapse. Several authors found no local relapses after total doses of 45 Gy. It has also been demonstrated that lower craniospinal doses 25-30 Gy will eradicate microscopic residual tumor, suggesting that the dose for both gross and microscopic residual tumor may be lowered without effecting the overall rate of disease control [73, 75, 76, 82, 85].

NGGCTs are relatively radioresistant and associated with a poor outcome ranging from 20 to 45% survival following neuraxis radiotherapy alone. The treatment of patients with intracranial NGGCT should be based on tumor histology. Treatment of patients who had a good prognosis (mature teratoma with germinoma) with surgical resection and radiotherapy was sufficient. Multimodal treatment of patients in the intermediate prognosis group, including surgical resection, radiotherapy and chemotherapy was effective. The choice of irradiation field in treatment of localized tumor remains unclear [86]. A high incidence of primary site failure highlights the need for more intensive chemotherapy or higher radiation doses to the primary tumor for patients with poor response to chemotherapy or radiation [81, 86, 87]. Several authors have advocated the use of prophylactic spinal irradiation in patients who have an intermediate or poor prognosis. They observed a 15-21% rate of spinal recurrence in patients who did not receive prophylactic spinal irradiation [85, 88].

Craniopharyngioma

Craniopharyngioma is benign tumor that arises from epithelial remnants of Rathke's pouch, and they constitute 2% to 9% of intracranial tumors in children [1]. Although these tumors are histologically benign, they are locally aggressive and invade adjacent critical structures like optic nerves, optic chiasm, pituitary gland, hypothalamus, third ventricle and blood vessels. There are two widely practiced treatment options: primary total resection and subtotal resection followed by external-beam radiotherapy. The goal of treatment in children with craniopharyngioma is to maximize local control and minimize acute and long-term treatment-related complications [3, 89-91]. Complete resection is achievable in 70-90% of cases and 60-80% remains relapse-free. However, forms that are incompletely resected will relapse in approximately 70% of cases. In children with recurrent craniopharyngioma after primary radical resection, the use of tree-dimensional conformal radiotherapy or fractionated stereotactic radiotherapy results in very good local control with a low incidence of complications. The use of secondary surgery for recurrent tumors is associated with all low cure rates and a high risk of complications [89, 90].

In most experts' opinions external radiation should be applied early in the treatment course and following limited surgical resection. External irradiation has been recommended following incomplete surgical resection or sometimes following a simple biopsy [89-92]. Total doses usually range between 45 and 55 Gy, with conventional fractionation. Five-year survival is in excess of 80% [89, 91]. Further improvement in the outcome might explore doses escalated above 55 Gy with stereotactic fractionated radiotherapy and optimal sparing of adjacent normal structures [9, 91].

Despite evidence that radiotherapy provides long-term disease control for most patients, there has been much concern about its potential impact on growth and development and on performance in school and at home. Because endocrine deficiencies are frequently induced by the tumor or by any treatment that precedes radiotherapy (i.e. surgery); radiation should not be avoided solely in an effort to prevent an endocrine deficit [90].

For many patients, radiotherapy may be favored as the primary treatment modality to avert the risk of visual impairment imposed by surgery.

In our Radiotherapy Department, in 1997-2001, 8 children with craniopharyngioma were treated with conformal radiotherapy techniques. All patients were referred to radiation due to recurrent tumor, after multiple surgeries. After median time of follow-up 48 months, all children are living with no recurrence (5) or with stable disease (3). We did not observe radiotherapy-related complications [20].

This is an agreement now, that limited surgery and radiotherapy cause lesser or comparable sequelae. Newer radiation planing and delivery techniques made a combined modality a good initial option for most patients with craniopharyngioma.

Conclusion

The modern radiotherapy techniques as conformal radiotherapy and stereotactic fractionated radiotherapy has been shown to be an appropriate treatment for many pediatric brain tumors.

For patients with low-grade astrocytomas, the first method of treatment is surgery. Radiotherapy is recommended as the treatment of choice in patients with inoperable or partially resected tumors with conventionally fractionated total dose 54 Gy. The radiotherapy target volume need include only the residual disease with small margin at the normal tissue.

Radiation therapy is a primary component of initial management of pediatric malignant glioma. The treatment volume should include the macroscopic preoperative tumor and 2 cm safety margin and with total doses at least 55-60 Gy.

The small proportion of patients with brain stem gliomas could be treated with surgery. For most patients (80%) with diffuse intrinsic brain stem tumors radiotherapy is treatment of choice. Current standard treatment consist to conventional radiotherapy, using local fields and doses of 54 Gy over 6 weeks, with one daily fraction.

Craniospinal radiotherapy is an essential component of the therapy of medulloblastoma with standard doses for whole CNS 35-36 Gy, followed by 18-20 Gy boost to primary tumor site. The primary tumor bed with 1-2 cm margin rather than whole posterior fossa should be included. The reduced doses for CNS with adjuvant chemotherapy for low-risk patients could be considered. The influence of quality of radiotherapy on treatment results is established, and CT - based 3-D treatment planning is mandatory.

The current recommendation for patients with ependymoma is to treat all supratentorial and low-grade infratentorial tumors with partial brain fields, encompassing the primary tumor bed with 2 cm margin, with doses $\geq$ 55 Gy. Craniospinal irradiation should be reserved for patients with evidence of craniospinal seeding.

The treatment of CNS germinoma should be based on a balanced assessment of the probability of tumor control and treatment related side effects. For young children, the chemotherapy, with limited - field and low - dose radiotherapy could be the best option. For older patients, especially for these with diabetes insipidus, the low-dose craniospinal radiotherapy with boost for primary tumor site could be considered.

For craniopharyngioma radiotherapy should be applied early in the treatment course, and following limited surgical resection. The use of 3-D conformal radiotherapy or fractionated stereotactic radiotherapy with doses 55 Gy results in very good local control, with a low incidence of complications.

The radiotherapy technique will be utilized is that which spares the greatest volume of normal tissue. With modern imaging modalities, CT simulation, image fusion and 3-D planning, as well as the availability of radiotherapy treatment equipment that allows the use of multiple, noncoplanar field arrangements, customized field shaping and intensity modulation of the radiation beam, conformity of the treatment volume to the target will easier to achieve. For small tumors (< 3-4 cm) fractionated stereotactic radiotherapy using multiple fixed non-coplanar beams will be an appropriate treatment. Modifications of craniospinal technique, lowering of the total craniospinal dose with adjuvant chemotherapy, new radiotherapy modalities to treat the posterior fossa and spinal fields (electrons, protons, intensity modulation radiation therapy) and hyperfractionated craniospinal radiotherapy may be employed to possibly decrease the late effects of radiation therapy. For malignant gliomas and brain stem tumors we need new approaches, as chemosensitization, angiogenesis inhibitors and gene therapies.

References

[1] Halperin, E; Constine, L; Tarbell, N; Kun, L. *Pediatric Radiation Oncology*. Third Edition. Philadelphia, USA: Lippincott Williams and Wilkins, 1999, 37-125.

[2] Merchant, TE; Zhu, Y; Thompson, SJ; et al. Preliminary results from a phase II trial of conformal radiation therapy for pediatric patients with localized low-grade astrocytoma and ependymoma. *Int J Radiat Oncol Biol Phys*, 2002 52, 325-332.

[3] Skowrońska-Gardas, A. Evaluation of radiotherapy for pediatric CNS tumors. *Expert Rev Neurotherapeutics*, 2003 3, 491-500.

[4] Loeffler, J; Kooy, H; Tarbell, N. The emergence of conformal radiotherapy: special implications for pediatric neuro-oncology. *Int J Radiat Oncol Biol Phys*,1999 44, 237-238.

[5] Skowrońska-Gardas, A; Morawska-Kaczyńska, M. Conformal radiotherapy in paediatric brain tumours. In: Monduzzi Editore. *Progress in Radio Oncology* VI. Bologna, Italy; 1998; 639-643.

[6] Svensson, H; Moller, TR. Developments in Radiotherapy. *Acta Oncologica*, 2003 42, 430-442.

[7] Jalali, R; Budrukkar, A; Sarin, R; et al. High precision conformal radiotherapy employing conservative margins in childhood benign and low-grade brain tumours. *Radiother Oncol*, 2005 74, 37-44.

[8] Brahme, A. Optimization of radiation therapy. *Int J Radiat Oncol Biol Phys*, 1994 28, 785-787.

[9] Adams, E; Suter, B; Warrington, A; et al. Design and implementation of a system for treating pediatric patients with stereotactically - guided conformal radiotherapy. *Radiother Oncol*, 2001 60, 289-297.

[10] Saran, FH; Baumert, BG; Khoo, VS; et al. Stereotactically guided conformal radiotherapy for progressive low-grade gliomas of childhood. *Int J Radiat Oncol Biol Phys*, 2002 53, 43-51.

[11] Marcus, KJ; Goumnerova, L; Billett, AL.; et al. Stereotactic radiotherapy for localized low-grade gliomas in children: final results of a prospective trial. *Int J Radiat Oncol Biol Phys*, 2005 61, 374-379.

[12] Murthy, V; Jalali, R; Sarin, R; et al. Stereotactic conformal radiotherapy for posterior fossa tumours: a modeling study for potential improvement in therapeutic ratio. *Radiother Oncol*, 2003 67, 191-198.

[13] Fukunaga-Johnson, N; Sandler, H; Marsh, R; et al. The use of 3 D conformal radiotherapy (3 D CRT) to spare the cochlea in patients with medulloblastoma. *Int J Radiat Oncol Biol Phys*,1998 41, 77-82.

[14] Paulino, AC; Narayama, A; Mohideen, MN; et al. Posterior fossa boost in medulloblastoma: an analysis of dose to surrounding structures using 3-dimensional (conformal) radiotherapy. *Int J Radiat Oncol Biol Phys*, 2000 46, 281-286.

[15] Hodgson, DC; Goumnerova, LC; Loeffler, JS; et al. Radiosurgery in management of pediatric brain tumors. *Int J Radiat Oncol Biol Phys*, 2001 50, 929-935.

[16] Lin, R; Hug, EB; Schaefer, RA; et al. Conformal proton radiation therapy of the posterior fossa: a study comparing protons with three-dimensional planned photons in limiting dose to auditory structures. *Int J Radiat Oncol Biol Phys*, 2000 48, 1219-1226.

[17] Tarbell, NJ; Smith, AR; Adams, J; et al. The challenge of conformal radiotherapy in the curative treatment of medulloblastoma. *Int J Radiat Oncol Biol Phys*, 2000 46, 265-266.

[18] Freeman, C; Farmer, JP; Montes, J. Low-grade astrocytomas in children: evolving management strategies. *Int J Radiat Oncol Biol Phys*,1998 41, 979-987.

[19] Kortmann, RD; Timmermann, B; Taylor, RE; et al. Current and future strategies in radiotherapy of childhood low-grade glioma of the brain. *Strahlenther Onkol*, 2003 179, 585-597.

[20] Skowrońska-Gardas, A; Chojnacka, M.; Pędziwiatr, K. Conformal radiotherapy in children with low-grade brain tumours: treatment results and toxicity. *Rep Pract Oncol Radiother*, 2005 10, 135-140.

[21] Campbell, JW; Pollock, JF; Martinez, AJ; et al. Radiologically complete resection is associated with excellent long-term prognosis. *Neurosurgery*, 1996 38, 258-264.

[22] Oppitz, U; Maessen, D; Zunterer, H; et al. 3-D recurrence-patterns of glioblastomas after CT-planned postoperative irradiation. *Radiother Oncol*, 1999 53, 53-57.

[23] Fallai, C; Olmi, P. Hyperfractionated and accelerated radiation therapy in central nervous system tumors (malignant gliomas, pediatric tumors and brain metastases). *Radiother Oncol*, 1997 43, 235-246.

[24] Pollack, I; Boyett, J; Finlay, J. Chemotherapy for high-grade gliomas of childhood. *Child's Nerv Syst*, 1999 15, 529-544.

[25] Freeman, CR; Farmer, JP. Pediatric brain stem gliomas: a review. *Int J Radiat Oncol Biol Phys*, 1998 40, 265-271.

[26] Schulz-Ertner, D; Debus, J; Lohr, F; et al. Fractionated stereotactic conformal radiation therapy of brain stem gliomas: outcome and prognostic factors. *Radiother Oncol*, 2000 57, 215-223.

[27] Donanue, B; Allen, J; Siffert, J; et al. Patterns of recurrence in brain stem gliomas: evidence for craniospinal dissemination. *Int J Radiat Oncol Biol Phys*, 1998 40, 677-680.

[28] Skowrońska-Gardas, A. Hyperfractionated radiotherapy for brain-stem tumors in children. *Radiother Oncol*, 1994 33, 259-261.

[29] Fischer, P; Donaldson, S. Hyperfractionated radiotherapy in the management of diffuse intrinsic brain stem tumors: when is enough? *Int J Radiat Oncol Biol Phys*, 1999 43, 947-949.

[30] Freeman, CR; Kepner, J; Kun, LE; et al. A detrimental effect of a combined chemotherapy - radiotherapy approach in children with diffuse intrinsic brain stem gliomas? *Int J Radiat Oncol Biol Phys*, 2000 47, 561-564.

[31] Mandell, L; Kadota, R; Freeman C; et al. There is no role for hyperfractionated radiotherapy in the management of children with newly diagnosed diffuse intrinsic brain stem tumors: results of a Pediatric Oncology Group phase III trial comparing conventional vs. hyperfractionated radiotherapy. *Int J Radiat Oncol Biol Phys*, 1999 43, 959-964.

[32] Allen, J; Siffert, J; Donahue, B; et al. A phase I/II study of carboplatin compiled with hyperfractionated radiotherapy for brainstem gliomas. *Cancer*,1999 86, 1064-1068.

[33] Bouffet, E; Raquin, M.; Doz, F; et al. Radiotherapy followed by high dose busulfan and thiotepa. A prospective assessment of high dose chemotherapy in children with diffuse pontine gliomas. *Cancer*, 2000 88, 685-692.

[34] Skowrońska-Gardas, A; Pędziwiatr, K; Chojnacka, M. Evaluation of quality of life in long-term survivors of paediatric brain stem tumors, treated with radiotherapy. *Radiother Oncol*, 2004 70, 269-273.

[35] Zeltzer, P.; Boyett, J; Finlay, J; et al. Metastasis stage, adjuvant treatment and residual tumor are prognostic factors for medulloblastoma in children: conclusions from the Children's Cancer Group 921 randomized phase III study. *J Clin Oncol*, 1999 17, 832-845.

[36] Kortmann, R; Kühl, J; Timmermann, P; et al. Postoperative neoadjuvant chemotherapy before radiotherapy as compared to immediate radiotherapy followed by maintenance chemotherapy in the treatment of medulloblastoma in childhood: results of the german prospective randomized trial HIT 91. *Int J Radiat Oncol Biol Phys*,2000 46, 269-279.

[37] Ris, D; Packer, R; Goldwein, J; et al. Intellectual outcome after reduced-dose radiation therapy plus adjuvant chemotherapy for medulloblastoma: a Children's Cancer Group Study. *J Clin Oncol*, 2001 19, 3470-3476.

[38] Packer, R; Goldwein, J; Nicholson, H; et al. Treatment of children with medulloblastoma with reduced - dose craniospinal radiation therapy and adjuvant chemotherapy: A Children's Cancer Group Study. *J Clin Oncol*, 1999 17, 2127-2136.

[39] Taylor, RE. United Kingdom Children's Cancer Study Group (UKCCSG) Radiotherapy and Brain Tumour Groups: Medulloblastoma/PNET and craniospinal radiotherapy (CSRT): report of a workshop held in Leeds, 30 June 1999. *Clinical Oncology*, 2001 13, 58-64.

[40] Ellison, DW; Clifford, SC; Gajjar, A; et al. What's new in neuro-oncology? Recent advances in medulloblastoma. *Eur J Pediatr Neurol*, 2003 7, 53-66.

[41] Freeman, C; Taylor, R; Kortmann, RD; et al. Radiotherapy for medulloblastoma in children: a prospective on current international clinical research efforts. *Med Ped Oncol*, 2002 39, 99-108.

[42] Charco, J; Bolek, T; McCollough, M.; et al. Medulloblastoma: time - dose relationship based on a 30-year review. *Int J Radiat Oncol Biol Phys*,1998 42, 147-154.

[43] Chojnacka, M; Skowrońska-Gardas, A. Medulloblastoma in childhood: impact of radiation technique upon the outcome of treatment. *Pediatr Blood Cancer*, 2004 42, 155-160.

[44] Kocsis, B; Szekely, G; Pap, L; et al. Effects of radiation treatment planning and patient fixation on the results of postoperative radiotherapy of childhood medulloblastoma. *Strahlenther Onkol*, 2003 179, 854-59.

[45] Halperin, E. Impact of radiation technique upon the outcome of treatment for medulloblastoma. *Int J Radiat Oncol Biol Phys*,1996 36, 233-239.

[46] Grabenauer, G; Beck, J; Erhardt, J; et al. Postoperative radiotherapy of medulloblastoma. Impact of radiation quality on treatment outcome. *Am J Clin Oncol*, 1996 19, 73-77.

[47] Miralbell, R; Bleher, A; Huegenin, P; et al. Pediatric medulloblastoma: radiation treatment technique and patterns of failure. *Int J Radiat Oncol Biol Phys*,1997 37, 523-529.

[48] Narayama, A; Jeswani, S; Paulino, A. The craniospinal junction in medulloblastoma: does it matter? *Int J Radiat Oncol Biol Phys*, 1999 44, 81-84.

[49] Scharf, C; Paulino, A; Goldberg, K. Determination of the inferior border of the thecal sac using magnetic resonance imaging: implications on radiation therapy treatment planning. *Int J Radiat Oncol Biol Phys*,1998 41, 621-624.

[50] Weiss, E; Krebek, M.; Kohler, B; et al. Does the standardized helmet technique lead to adequate coverage of the cribriform plate? An analysis of current practice with respect of the ICRU 50 report. *Int J Radiat Oncol Biol Phys*, 2001 49, 1475-1480.

[51] Wolden, SL; Dunkel, IJ; Souweidane, MM; et al. Patterns of failure using a conformal radiation therapy tumor bed boost for medulloblastoma. *J Clin Oncol*, 2003 21, 3079-3083.

[52] Jereb, B; Krishnaswami, S; Reid, A: et al. Radiation for medulloblastoma adjusted to prevent recurrence to the cribriform plate region. *Cancer*, 1984 54, 602-604.

[53] Carrie, C; Alapetite, C; Mere, P; et al. Quality control of radiotherapeutic treatment of medulloblastoma in a multicentric study: The contribution of radiotherapy technique to tumor relapse. *Radiother Oncol*, 1992 24, 77-81.

[54] Mc Laughin, M.; Marcus, R; Buatti, J; et al. Ependymoma: results, prognostic factors and treatment recommendation. *Int J Radiat Oncol Biol Phys*, 1998 40, 845-850.

[55] Schild, S; Nisi, K; Scheithaur, B; et al. The results or radiotherapy for ependymomas: the Mayo Clinic experience. *Int J Radiat Oncol Biol Phys*, 1998 42, 953-958.

[56] Timmermann, B; Kortmann, R; Kühl, J; et al. Combined postoperative irradiation and chemotherapy for anaplastic ependymomas in childhood: results on the german prospective trials HIT 88/89 and HIT 91. *Int J Radiat Oncol Biol Phys*, 2000 46, 287-295.

[57] Healey, EA; Braners, PD; Kupley, WJ; et al. The prognostic significance of postoperative residual tumor in ependymoma. *Neurosurgery*,1991 28, 666-672.

[58] Massimino, M.; Gandola, L; Giangaspero, F; et al. Hyperfractionated radiotherapy and chemotherapy for childhood ependymoma: final results of the first prospective AIEOP (Associazione Italiana di Ematologia-Oncologia Pediatrica) study. *Int J Radiat Oncol Biol Phys*, 2004 58, 1336-1345.

[59] Merchant, TE; Jenkins, JJ; Burger, PC; et al. Influence of tumor grade on time to progression after irradiation for localized ependymoma in children. *Int J Radiat Oncol Biol Phys*, 2002 53, 52-57.

[60] Robertson, PL; Zeltzer, PM; Boyett, JM; et al. Prognostic factors following radiation therapy and chemotherapy for ependymomas in children: a report of the Children's Cancer Group. *J Neurosurg*, 1998 88, 695-703.

[61] Mansur, DB; Perry, A; Rajaram, V; et al. Postoperative radiation therapy for grade II and III intracranial ependymoma. *Int J Radiat Oncol Biol Phys*, 2005 61, 387-391.

[62] Carrie, C; Mottolese, C; Bouffet, E; et al. Non-metastatic childhood ependymoma. *Radiother Oncol*, 1995 36, 101-106.

[63] Kovalic, JJ; Flaris, N; Grigsby, PW; et al. Intracranial ependymoma long-term outcome, patterns of failure. *J Neurooncol*, 1993 15, 125-131.

[64] Goldwein, JW; Corn, BW; Finlay, JL; et al. Is craniospinal irradiation required to cure children with malignant (anaplastic) intracranial ependymomas? *Cancer*, 1991 67, 2766-2771.

[65] Rousseau, P; Habrand, J; Sarrazin, D; et al. Treatment of intracranial ependymomas of children: review of a 15-year experience. *Int J Radiat Oncol Biol Phys*, 1994 28, 381-386.

[66] Paulino, AC; B-Chen Wen. The significance of radiotherapy treatment duration in intracranial ependymoma. *Int J Radiat Oncol Biol Phys*, 2000 47, 585-589.

[67] Paulino, AC. The local field in infratentorial ependymoma: does the entire posterior fossa need to be treated? *Int J Radiat Oncol Biol Phys*, 2001 49, 757-761.

[68] Merchant, TE; Haida, T; Wang, MH; et al. Anaplastic ependymoma: treatment of pediatric patients with or without craniospinal radiation therapy. *J Neurosurg*, 1997 86, 943-949.

[69] Duffner, PK; Horowitz, ME; Krischer, JP; et al. Postoperative chemotherapy and delayed radiation in children less than 3 yeas of age with malignant brain tumors. *N Engl J Med*, 1993 328, 1725-1731.

[70] Evans, AE; Anderson, JR; Lefkowitz-Boudreaux, IB; et al. Craniospinal irradiation with or without adjuvant CCNU, vincristine, and prednisone: A Children Cancer Group study. *Med Pediatr Oncol*, 1996 27, 8-14.

[71] Merchant, TE; Mulhern, RK; Krasin, MJ; et al. Preliminary results from a phase II trial of conformal radiation therapy and evaluation of radiation-related CNS effects for pediatric patients with localized ependymoma. *J Clin Oncol*, 2004 22, 3156-3162.

[72] Hoffman, HJ; Otsubo, H; Hendrick, EB; et al. Intracranial germ-cell tumors in children. *J Neurosurg*, 1991 74, 545-551.

[73] Haas-Kogan, DA; Missett, BT; Wara, WM; et al. Radiation therapy for intracranial germ cell tumors. *Int J Radiat Oncol Biol Phys*, 2003 56, 511-518.

[74] Wolden, SL; Wara, WM; Larson, DA; et al. Radiation therapy for primary intracranial germ cell tumors. *Int J Radiat Oncol Biol Phys*, 1995 32, 943-949.

[75] Merchant, T; Sherwood, S; Mulhern, R; et al. CNS germinoma: disease control and long-term functional outcome for 12 children treated with craniospinal irradiation. *Int J Radiat Oncol Biol Phys*, 2000 46, 1171-1176.

[76] Ogawa, K; Shikama, N; Toita, T; et al. Long-term results of radiotherapy for intracranial germinoma: a multi-institutional retrospective review of 126 patients. *Int J Radiat Oncol Biol Phys*, 2004 58, 705-713.

[77] Maity, A; Shu, G; Janss, A; et al. Craniospinal radiation in the treatment of biopsy-proven intracranial germinomas: twenty-five years' experience in a single center. *Int J Radiat Oncol Biol Phys*, 2004 58, 1165-1170.

[78] Bouffet, E; Baranzelli, M; Patte, C; et al. Combined treatment modality for intracranial germinomas: results of a multicentre SFOP experience. *Br J Cancer*, 1999 79, 1199-1204.

[79] Aoyama, H; Shirato, H; Ikeda, J; et al. Induction chemotherapy followed by low-dose involved-field radiotherapy for intracranial germ cell tumors. *J Clin Oncol*, 2002 20, 857-865.

[80] Shirato, H; Aoyama, H; Ikeda, J; et al. Impact of margin for target volume in low-dose involved field radiotherapy after induction chemotherapy for intracranial germinoma. *Int J Radiat Oncol Biol Phys*, 2004 60, 214-217.

[81] Matsutani, M; Sano, K; Takakura, K; et al. Primary intracranial germ cell tumors: a clinical analysis of 153 histologically verified cases. *J Neurosurg*, 1997 86, 446-455.

[82] Shibamoto, Y; Abe, M; Yamashita, J; et al. Treatment results of intracranial germinoma as a function of the irradiated volume. *Int J Radiat Oncol Biol Phys*, 1988 15, 285-290.

[83] Dattoli, MJ; Newall, J. Radiation therapy for intracranial germinoma: the case for limited volume treatment. *Int J Radiat Oncol Biol Phys*, 1990 19, 429-433.

[84] Alapetite, C; Ricardi, U; Saran, F; et al. Whole ventricular irradiation in combination with chemotherapy in intracranial germinoma: the consensus of the SIOP CNS CGT study group. *Med Pediatr Oncol*, 2002 39, 248.

[85] Shirato, H; Nishio, M; Sawamura, Y; et al. Analysis of long term treatment of intracranial germinoma. *Int J Radiat Oncol Biol Phys*, 1997 37, 511-515.

[86] Ogawa, K; Toita, T; Nakamura, K; et al. Treatment and prognosis of patients with intracranial nongerminomatous malignant germ cell tumors. *Cancer*, 2003 98, 369-376.

[87] Kellie, SJ; Boyce, H; Dunkel, IJ; et al. Primary chemotherapy for intracranial nongerminomatous germ cell tumors: results of the Second International CNS Germ Cell Study Group Protocol. *J Clin Oncol*, 2004 22, 846-853.

[88] Aoyama, H; Shirato, H; Yoshida, H; et al. Retrospective multiinstitutional study of radiotherapy for intracranial non-germinomatous germ cell tumors. *Radiother Oncol*, 1998 49, 55-59.

[89] Kalapurakel, JA; Goldman, S; Hsieh, YC; et al. Clinical outcome in children with recurrent craniopharyngioma after primary surgery. *Cancer J*, 2000 6, 388-393.

[90] Merchant, TE; Kiehna, EN; Sanford, RA; et al. Craniopharyngioma: The St. Jude Children's Research Hospital experience 1984-2001. *Int J Radiat Oncol Biol Phys*, 2002 53, 533-542.

[91] Habrand, JL; Ganry, O; Couanet, D; et al. The role of radiation therapy in the management of craniopharyngioma: a 25-year experience and review of the literature. *Int J Radiat Oncol Biol Phys*, 1999 44, 255-263.

[92] Khafaga, Y; Jenkin, D; Kanaau, I; et al. Craniopharyngioma in children. *Int J Radiat Oncol Biol Phys*,1998 42, 601-606.

In: Brain Cancer Therapy and Surgical Interventions... ISBN 1-59454-974-5
Editor: Andrew V. Yang, pp. 147-169

Chapter VII

Stereotactic Radiosurgery/ Radiotherapy in the Management of Low Grade Gliomas

David Roberge,[1] Luis Souhami,[1] André Olivier,[2] Richard Leblanc[2] and Ervin Porgorsak[3]

[1]Department of Oncology, Division of Radiation Oncology, McGill University, Montreal, Canada

[2]Department of Neurosurgery, Montreal Neurological Institute, McGill University, Montreal, Canada

[3]Department of Medical Physics, McGill University, Montreal, Canada

Abstract

Primary brain tumors are classified according to their predominant cell type. According to the Central Brain Tumor Registry of the United States (CBTRUS), glial neoplasms are the most common primary intracranial malignancies. Although the use of SRS for well-defined small low-grade tumors is appealing, the data regarding the use of SRS is limited and insufficient to support a standard role for SRS in the initial management of low-grade gliomas. The technologies of F-SRT will slowly be integrated into conventional therapy, treatment margins will be reduced and SRS will be limited to very selected recurrent tumors.

Introduction

Primary brain tumors are classified according to their predominant cell type. According to the Central Brain Tumor Registry of the United States (CBTRUS), glial neoplasms are the most common primary intracranial malignancies [1]. They can be classified as astrocytic, oligodendroglial or ependymal tumors. Each of these tumor groups is further subdivided by grade, with tumors of grade I and II referred to as low-grade. The WHO classification of these tumors is presented in Table 1.

Table 1: WHO classification of low-grade glial tumors [104]

Astrocytic tumors	
Grade I	Pilocytic Astrocytoma
	Subependymal giant cell astrocytoma
Grade II	Diffuse astrocytoma
	Fibrillary astrocytoma
	Protoplasmic astrocytoma
	Gemistocytic astrocytoma
	Pleomorphic xanthoastrocytoma
Oligodendroglial tumors	
Grade II	Oligodendroglioma
Mixed gliomas	
Grade II	Oligoastrocytoma
Ependymal tumors	
Grade I	Myxopapillary ependymoma
	Subependymoma
Grade II	Ependymoma
	Cellular
	Papillary
	Clear cell
	Tanycytic

In incidence, high-grade tumors outnumber their low-grade counterparts, as glioblastoma multiforme is by far the most common tumor of neuroepithelial origin. Overall, only 5 to 10% of gliomas are low-grade lesions. In the pediatric population the ratio of incidence is reversed — pilocytic astrocytomas outnumbering all other glial neoplasms [2].

Prognostic Factors

Patients with low-grade gliomas form a very heterogeneous population. At opposite ends of the clinical spectrum, pediatric patients with cerebellar pilocytic astrocytomas can expect 90% 10-year survival [2-5], whereas patients over 40 with a poor performance status face a dismal 50% 1-year overall survival [6]. Prognostic factors have been examined in numerous retrospective series [5-19]. Prognostic factors identified relate to histologic, imaging and morphologic tumor features, to patient characteristics, as well as to treatment specific factors. In adults, the strongest prognostic features appear to be patient related — namely age, and measures of mental, neurological or functional status [6, 10].

In a multi-institutional retrospective review, prognostic groups were created for adult low-grade gliomas [6]. The prognostic factors retained by recursive partitioning analysis were: age, performance status and contrast enhancement on imaging studies. Using these factors, patients are divided into 4 groups with median survivals ranging from 12 months to 128 months (Table 2). Despite the apparent ability of this simple prognostic scheme to define groups with large clinically and statistically significant differences in outcome, the scheme has not gained the widespread acceptance of the recursive partitioning scheme used for high-grade gliomas [20, 21].

Table 2: Prognostic groups for adult Grade II gliomas defined by recursive partitioning analysis [6]

Prognostic group	Median overall survival
Group I Karnofsky performance status < 70 Age > 40	12 months
Group II Karnofsky performance status ≥ 70 Age > 40 Presence of contrast enhancement	46 months
Group III Karnofsky performance status < 70 Age 18-40 *Or* Karnofsky performance status ≥ 70 Age > 40 Absence of contrast enhancement	87 months
Group IV Karnofsky performance status ≥ 70 Age 18-40	128 months

Pertinent to any review of radiosurgical treatments is the prognostic influence of target size. As radiosurgical series invariably exclude tumors based on size, they will be prone to bias in any disease where tumor volume is of prognostic consequence. Unfortunately, because the information was not present in all three retrospective series used, volume was not included in the recursive partitioning analysis model. However, in a multivariate analysis of data from 322 patients (validated on a second set of 288 patients), Pignatti et al. [10] have shown largest tumor diameter ≥ 6 cm to be a poor prognostic factor. Median overall survival was 3.52 years for patients with larger tumors compared to 8.02 years for patients with tumors < 6 cm (HR 1.43, $p = 0.0001$). In an analysis of 203 patients, Shaw et al. [22] have shown tumor size ≥ 5 cm to convey a poor prognosis with a 5-year overall survival of 61% vs. 81% for smaller tumors ($p = 0.0008$). In a series of smaller tumors (0.5-70 cc) treated with interstitial brachytherapy, tumor volume > 20 cm [3] was, on multivariate analysis, associated with a worse prognosis (RR 1.9, $p < 0.02$) [23]. The prognostic impact of tumor size is also seen in the pediatric population where, in a prospective trial, residual tumor greater than 3 cm^3 was strongly associated with worse progression-free and overall survival [24].

Current Therapy

Despite the lack of Class I evidence [25, 26], the primary management of low-grade gliomas is maximal safe resection [27, 28]. Although this may be debated in adults with unfavorable pretreatment characteristics, the standard of care following gross total resection is observation. In children this strategy leads to long-term disease-free and overall survival of 80 to 100% [24, 28-32]. In adults, gross total resection has been reported to be associated with wide ranging 5-year survival figures — 51 to 100% [7, 26, 33-37]. The most controversial area in the management of low-grade gliomas has been the use of adjuvant therapy following an incomplete surgical resection. In the adult population, two randomized trials have failed to demonstrate a survival advantage to the addition of CCNU [38] or PCV [39] to standard external beam radiotherapy. Thus, despite high response rates in selected patients with oligodendroglial tumors [40, 41], chemotherapy is generally reserved for unresectable post-radiotherapy progression. In infants, where delaying the use of radiotherapy may be of value, chemotherapy has a larger role [28]. In a series of hypothalamic/chiasmatic region tumors, 72% of patients eventually progressed post-chemotherapy but radiotherapy was successfully delayed beyond age 5 in more than 70% of cases [42].

The main focus of controversy regarding the adjuvant treatment of low-grade gliomas has centered on the use of radiotherapy. In 1968, Dr Arthur R. Elvidge, working at the Montreal Neurological Institute wrote "The majority of piloid tumors in long-term survivors contained cysts. The effect of x-ray therapy is difficult to evaluate and is certainly of doubtful benefit for the piloid types." "In gemistocytic astrocytomas, long-term survival is limited. Of 21 patients [...] only 2 reached 10 years. X-ray therapy did not seem to be very effective in this group, although it should nevertheless be recommended because of its known beneficial effect in the closely related glioblastoma multiforme" [43]. Dr. Jean Bouchard, then professor of radiology at McGill university and contemporary of Penfield and Elvidge, wrote in his 1966 textbook: "Technically, we presently treat cerebral astrocytomas postoperatively with Cobalt [60] high energy radiation by delivering tumor doses averaging 5000 to 6000 rads over a period of 45 to 50 days [...] The evidence presented above strongly indicates that supratentorial astrocytomas arising in the cerebral hemispheres can be treated best by surgical removal combined with postoperative irradiation. Comparative survival rates strongly suggest that beyond the third year after treatment, longevity is increasingly greater among patients who had postoperative irradiation than in those treated solely by surgery." [44] Until recently such evidence, based on case series, was all that clinicians could rely upon in making treatment decisions regarding the application of therapeutic radiation.

In the past decade, 3 randomized trials have been published in regards to adjuvant radiotherapy. Two trials failed to show a radiotherapeutic dose-response for the dose levels studied. In both the EORTC 22844 [45] randomizing patients between 45 Gy and 59.4 Gy and the Intergroup trial [22] comparing 50.4 Gy to 64.8 Gy, no difference in progression-free survival was seen. The third trial, EORTC 22845 [46] evaluated 54 Gy of external beam radiotherapy versus observation. In fact this became a trial of early vs. delayed radiotherapy as 60% of the patients in the control arm were eventually treated with radiotherapy at time of progression. The results were disappointing with adjuvant radiation conferring only a small advantage in 5-year progression-free survival (44% vs. 37%, $p = 0.02$) and time to progression (4.8 vs. 3.4 years). Early treatment had no impact on overall survival. The controversy thus continues [47] as radiation "believers" see an advantage in progression-free survival and "non-believers", the lack of impact on overall survival.

Radiosurgery

It was several decades following the introduction of the concept of stereotactic radiosurgery (SRS) by Leksell at the Karolinska institute in the early 1950s [48], that stereotactic irradiation began seeing widespread use in the treatment of brain tumors. In the management of gliomas most of the attention has been turned towards high-grade lesions [49]. The initial rationale for SRS in high-grade gliomas was founded on the poor clinical prognosis [21], the localized pattern of failure [50] and the initially promising results from interstitial brachytherapy series [51, 52]. Initial series with both gamma knife and linear accelerator-based treatments were promising with papers bearing titles such as: "Survival benefit of stereotactic radiosurgery for patients with malignant glial neoplasms" [53]. A debate began as to the biases of these retrospective series [54, 55], concerns subsequently justified by the negative results of a randomized RTOG trial [56]. The reality is that high grade gliomas make poor targets for SRS because they are acute-responding [57], uncontrolled by surgical excision and admixed with normal tissue [58, 59]. Except for selected cases of localized post-radiotherapy recurrences, enthusiasm for SRS in the treatment of high-grade gliomas has severely waned.

There may be a biologic rationale for low-grade gliomas being more appropriate SRS targets. Low-grade gliomas may be less infiltrative and have a lower α/β ratio [60] than their high-grade counterparts. They lack a dose-response relationship to increasing doses of external-beam radiotherapy. In these slow growing tumors, SRS may be therapeutic through the obliteration of tumor vasculature rather than through direct cytotoxicity [61].

When, in 1985, Colombo et al. [62] reported on the first patients treated with a new technique for linear accelerator-based SRS, the rationale cited was: (a) the bloodless nature of the treatment, (b) the convenience of these short treatment sessions and (c) the sparing of surrounding structures. In this initial publication from Vicenza, Italy only 6 patients had adequate follow-up. Of these, three patients were treated for low-grade gliomas. A 14 year-old with a left thalamic grade I astrocytoma was given two doses of 25 Gy during separate procedures, 17 months later the lesion had reduced in size. A 27 year-old with a right thalamic grade II ependymoma was given a similar treatment with reduction in size of his lesion, from 4 cm to 3.5 cm over the following 6 months. The third patient, a 56 year-old with a recurrent left thalamic oligodendroglioma had a stable lesion after 6 months of follow-up.

Table 3: Results of SRS or F-SRT in low-grade gliomas

Authors	Pozza et al. [63]	Barcia et al. [64]	Kida et al. [65]	Regine et al. [105]	Hadjipanayis at al. [66-68]	Boethius et al. [69]	Simonova et al. [70]	Souhami et al.
Center	Vicenza	Valencia	Komaki	Kentucky	Pittsburgh	Karolinska	Prague	McGill
Date of publication	1989	1994	2000	2000	2002	2002	2005	
Number of patients	14	16	51	5	49	19	70	21
Age (median)	16	20 (4-68)	9.8 Astro I* 30.9 Astro II*	≥18	14 Astro I 25 Astro II	10.6 (2-60)	17 (3-42)	27
Histology	Astro I/II	7 path. Confirmed Gr I/II	12 Astro I 39 Astro II	ASTRO II	37 Astro I 12 Astro II	Astro I	34 Astro I 34 Astro I/II	Mixed
Median Size (mm)	20	33 (15-50)	25.4 Astro I* 23.7 Astro II*	—	$3cm^3$ Astro I $4.6cm^3$ Astro II	$2.2cm^3$ (0.3-11.5)	$4.2cm^3$ (0.4-20)	14 (6-23)
Dose (Gy) / Fractions (#)	16-50/1-2	21.7/1 + EBRT 53.1 in 1.8-2Gy/day (0-66)	12.5/1 Astro I* 15.7/1 Astro II*	14/2 – 28/4 + 59.4/33 EBRT	15/1 Astro I 16/1 Astro II	10/1 (9-20/1)	25/5 (25-30)	37.5-45.5/6
Location	—	Brainstem 5 Thalamus 4 Other 7	—	—	Supratentorial 22 Optic tract 1 Brainstem 22 Cerebellum 4	Brainstem 12 Cerebellum 3 Supratentorial 4	—	See Table 4
Response Rate	85.5	50 CR	58 Astro I (PD in 8%) 62 Astro II (PD in 13%)	80 (partial or minor)	48 Astro I 42 Astro II	85 ("moderate" reduction)	83 (PR or CR)	14
Follow-up (months)	27.5	50 (5-156)	27.6*	43	28 Astro I 52 Astro II	84	≥48 months	132 (at risk 160)
Toxicity (%)	14	—	55	—	8 (clinical) Astro I 0 Astro II	25 (radiological)	7 (moderate-severe)	14
Survival	—	81% 10yr	—	80% 5yr	— Astro I 100% 5yr Astro II	100% 5yr	77 months median	76% 5yr 63% 15yr

ASTRO = astrocytoma
PD = progressive disease
PR = partial response
CR = complete response
* mean

Following the publication of this small series, several other centers have compiled their results in treating low-grade gliomas with SRS and fractionated stereotactic radiotherapy (F-SRT). In the following sections we will present these results (Table 3) as well as part of our own experience in this domain. We will attempt to offer pertinent commentary on the past and present as well as an outlook for the future of these therapeutic modalities in the management of low-grade gliomas.

Stereotactic Radiosurgery

Case Series

Adding 11 patients to the initial 3 presented in the 1985 series from Vicenza [62], Pozza et al. [63] published in 1989 a series of low grade gliomas treated with 1-2 fractions of stereotactic radiation. Five patients were treated with a single dose (16-20 Gy) and the other 10 with two fractions (8-25 Gy each) delivered with a one-week interval. Patients were treated at a median age of 16 (11-30) for small (7-25 mm) histologically verified grade I or II tumors. Tumor shrinkage was seen in 11 patients (74.6%). In 8 patients transient increase was seen in the apparent tumor — a phenomenon that reached its peak at a median of 4.5 months. With a short median follow-up of 27.5 months, one patient had treatment failure and died of progressive tumor growth 38 months following the procedure. Acute toxicity was seen in five patients, including the two patients treated with a total of 50 Gy.

In 1994, Barcia et al. [64] published a series of 16 patients treated between 1978 and 1991. Radiosurgery was delivered using a modified conventional Co [60] teletherapy unit. All patients were considered to have deep-seated low-grade gliomas, histologically confirmed in only 7 cases. In 12 patients, the SRS was given a median of 9 months after 42-66 Gy of external beam radiotherapy (1.8-2 Gy per fraction). The other 4 patients were treated with exclusive SRS (25-35 Gy). At a median follow-up of 50 months, the 10-year actuarial survival was 81%. In eight cases a radiological complete response was seen, in 2 a reduction in size, in 3 stabilization and in 3, progression. No serious complications were seen due to acute post-irradiation toxicity. Of note in this series are the high complete response rate, the absence of toxicity despite high delivered doses (as an example, the 8th patient in the series received 54 Gy of external beam radiotherapy through 4 ports followed by a 30 Gy SRS boost for a brainstem tumor) and an apparently unusual technique. As far as tumor response, four of the 8 complete responders lacked a histological diagnosis and it is not reported what proportion of the responding patients had undergone magnetic resonance imaging. The lack of observed toxicity might be related to the small size of the series and the fact that small circular collimators were used (5-10 mm, 1-2 isocenters). Regarding the technique, it appears that 81% of patients were treated with a single 10 mm collimator even though the smallest tumor had a maximal diameter of 15 mm (15-55). It is interesting that despite the favorable results presented in this series, there has been no update presenting further patients treated with this approach.

In 2000, Kida et al. [65] published a large series of patients treated at the Komaki City Hospital. Since 1991, 51 patients with low-grade astrocytomas had been treated with SRS.

Thirty-nine patients were treated for grade II astrocytomas, 12 for grade I astrocytomas located in and around the optic pathways and hypothalamus. The mean age was 9.8 years for grade I tumors and 30.9 for grade II tumors. With a short mean follow-up of 27.6 months, tumor control was good for both grade I and II tumors, 91.7% and 87.2%, respectively. Six patients had a complete response and 18 a partial response. The most common toxicity was radiation-induced edema (18 patients). Cyst formation, cyst progression, hydrocephalus and temporary tumor swelling were also seen.

In 2002, Hadjipanayis et al. [66] published the results of 37 patients treated for pilocytic astrocytomas at the University of Pittsburgh. These patients were treated over a 13-year period from 1987 to 2000. As is typical of this disease, the patients were young — 68% younger than 18 years of age. Tumors were both supratentorial (43%) and infratentorial (57%). All diagnoses had been pathologically confirmed and 24% of patients had undergone prior external beam radiotherapy. The cyst wall, if present, was included in the target volume. Median dose to the tumor margin was 15 Gy. The 7-year actuarial survival rate was 76%. Forty-nine percent of patients had a radiological response (complete in more than half) and 32% progressed. However, the actuarial 7-year failure rate was approximately 80%. As expected, age was a strong prognostic factor with a 100% actuarial 6-year failure rate in adults. Two patients experienced temporary worsening of their neurological condition and one required a VP shunt. In a 2003 update, it was reported that no patient had experienced late morbidity or mortality from the treatment [67].

A separate publication described a series of 12 patients treated for grade II astrocytomas at the University of Pittsburgh [68]. These patients were treated over a 13-year interval from 1987 to 2000. Seven were treated in the adjuvant setting following incomplete resection, 5 for failure of previous treatment. Median age was 25 years (range 5-57). These small tumors (0.9-45.1 cm^3) were treated with a median peripheral dose of 15 Gy (range 12-20 Gy). Four patients had brainstem tumors, 1 was in the cerebellum and the remaining seven were supratentorial. At a median follow-up of 52 months, all patients were alive. Radiological response was seen in 5 patients including one complete response. Three patients had cyst progression and one had solid tumor progression. No procedure related morbidity or mortality was reported. These results are promising but the fact that less than one patient per year was treated at this large radiosurgery practice is a sign of the limited numbers of patients felt to be appropriate candidates for this treatment and the important selection biases of such series.

In 2002, Boethius et al. [69] published a series of patients treated with SRS over a 19-year period (1978-1997) at the Karolinska hospital in Stockholm. These 19 patients were all treated for histologically confirmed pilocytic tumors. As would be expected for this histology, this was a predominantly pediatric population (median age 10.6 years, range 2-60). Twelve of the 19 tumors were located in the brainstem. Relatively low peripheral doses were used, generally 10-12 Gy (range 9-20 Gy) with corresponding maximal doses of 22-30 Gy (range 10-50 Gy). With a median clinical follow-up of 7 years, tumor control was achieved in all but one patient (cyst development occurred in 2 patients and was not considered treatment failure by the authors). In 85% of patients, tumor volume reduction was seen with a complete response in 4 cases. Radiation effect characterized by radiological appearance of transient edema and increased tumor enhancement was seen in 25% of patients, typically within 7 months of SRS. One patient underwent surgery for radionecrosis. As with the University of Pittsburgh series, the slow rate of accrual in the large center is evidence of the highly selected nature of these cases. This must be kept in mind in interpreting these favorable results.

In 2005, Simonova et al. published a series of 70 patients treated with a mix of gamma knife SRS and F-SRT using rigid immobilisation [70]. These patients were accrued over a relatively short 6-year period. They were young patients (median 17 years of age) with small (median 4.2 cm^3) histologically verified low-grade tumors. Half of the patients had grade I tumors and the remaining cases were graded as I/II. Seven patients were treated with SRS and 61 F-SRT. A quarter of these patients had received prior external beam radiotherapy. The typical prescription in this series was 25 Gy given in 5 daily fractions. Partial or complete tumor regression was seen in 83% of patients (excluding two patients lost to follow-up). The median time to local response was 18 months. With a minimum follow-up in living patients of 48 months, 5-year progression-free survival was 88%. Moderate to severe late toxicity was seen in 7% of patients.

McGill Experience

In conventional radiotherapy for tumors, fractionation is used to exploit the differential effect of fraction size on tumors and late reacting tissues. In considering SRS for low-grade gliomas, we were stimulated by the promising results obtained in the treatment of arteriovenous malformations and selected benign lesions as well as by SRS's characteristically sharp dose fall-off. However, we were concerned by the prospect of delivering large single doses of radiation to vital brain structures. In contrast to radiosurgery for other benign brain lesions, the treatment of potentially infiltrative tumors generally requires larger treatment volumes to include the tumor in its entirety with a "minimal safe margin". In addition to sparing normal brain, the use of fractionation may be advantageous in allowing reoxygenation of resistant, hypoxic, tumor cells and reassortment of tumor cells in less sensitive phases of the cell cycle (two of the 4 classic "R"s of radiobiology). These were the motivations for our 1987 initiation of a program of hypofractionated stereotactic radiotherapy for selected patients with low-grade gliomas. We were attempting to combine the radiobiological advantages of fractionation with the steep dose fall-off characteristics offered by SRS techniques.

From July 1987 to November 1992, 21 patients were treated at our institution using a hypofractionated regimen of stereotactic radiotherapy. Stringent selection criteria were used to offer patients this treatment regimen. All patients had well-circumscribed, < 4 cm, histologically proven, low-grade glial tumors. Patients were assessed by a team comprised of a radiation oncologist, a neurosurgeon, a neuroradiologist and a physicist. Lesions involved sensitive brain structures and were deemed unresectable. The patients treated with this technique were young (9-74, median 23 years of age) and predominantly female (60%). More patient characteristics are presented in Table 4.

Table 4: Patient characteristics, McGill LGG FSRT experience

Patient no.	Age (yr)	Sex	Histology	Tumor location
1	45	F	Astrocytoma NOS	Frontal
2	32	F	Astrocytoma GR II	Midbrain
3	9	F	Astrocytoma GR I	Lenticular
4	24	M	Astrocytoma GR I	Midbrain
5	38	M	Astrocytoma GR I	Midbrain
6	16	M	Astrocytoma GR II	Midbrain
7	37	F	Subependymoma	Pons
8	23	M	Oligoastrocytoma	Parietal
9	11	F	Astrocytoma GR I	Thalamus
10	22	F	Astrocytoma GR II	Pons
11	21	F	Astrocytoma GR II	Periventricu lar
12	74	M	Subependymoma	4th ventricle
13	13	M	Astrocytoma GR II	Thalamus
14	28	F	Astrocytoma Gr I-II (ganglioglioma on post-SRS resection)	Parietal
15	28	M	Astrocytoma GR II	Central
16	20	F	Astrocytoma GR II	Parietal
17	10	F	Astrocytoma GR II	Septum pellucidum
18	27	M	Astrocytoma GR II	4th ventricle
19	22	F	Astrocytoma GR II	Parietal
20	64	F	Astrocytoma GR II	Parietal
21	19	M	Astrocytoma GR II	Parietal

Irradiation targets were located by CT scanning and magnetic resonance imaging using a locally developed stereotactic frame [71, 72]. Following the first fraction the target information was tattooed onto the skin of the patient and the stereotactic frame was replaced with an immobilization halo ring affixed to the patient's skull (Figure II) [73]. The halo ring then remained in place for the duration of the treatment.

The stereotactic irradiation was delivered through the use of 10-40 mm circular cones (1-3 isocenters) using the McGill dynamic stereoctactic technique [73-75]. All treatments were delivered using a Varian Clinac 18 10 MV linear accelerator. Tumor doses ranged from 36 Gy to 46 Gy (median 42 Gy) in 6-7 fractions (median 6) of 5-7 Gy (median 7 Gy). The dose was typically prescribed to the 90% isodose surface encompassing the lesion with a 2 mm margin. Treatments were delivered on alternating days over a 2-week period. Technical parameters are given in Table 5.

Table 5: Technical parameters of fractionated treatments delivered at McGill

Patient no.	Number of isocenters	Cone diameter (mm)	Prescription isodose (%)	Total Dose (cGy)	Dose per fraction (cGy)	Number of fractions
1	1	30	80	4200	700	6
2	1	20	75	4600	500/600/700	7
3	1	15	87	4200	700	6
4	1	15	80	4200	700	6
5	1	20	74	4200	700	6
6	3	10/15/20	79	4300	600/700	7
7	1	25	72	4200	700	6
8	1	20	83	4200	700	6
9	1	15	75	4200	700	6
10	1	15	70	4200	700	6
11	1	20	76	4200	700	6
12	1	25	78	4200	700	6
13	1	40	68	3600	600	6
14	1	25	90	4200	700	6
15	1	40	90	4200	700	6
16	1	40	90	4200	700	6
17	1	22.5	90	3900	650	6
18	1	40	90	4200	700	6
19	1	25	90	4200	700	6
20	1	30	90	4200	700	6
21	1	35	90	4200	700	6

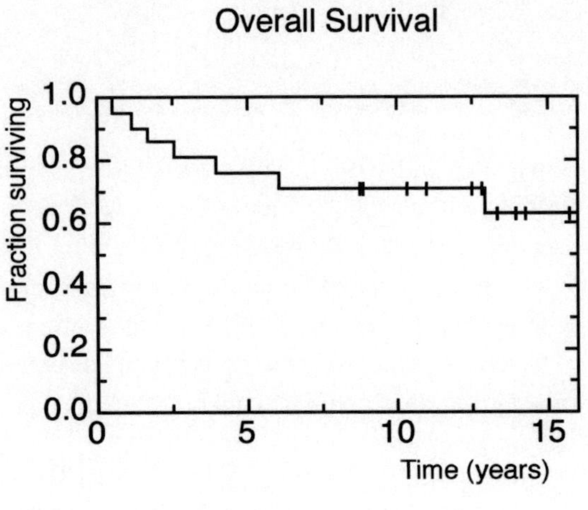

Figure 1: Overall survival following F-SRT at McGill University

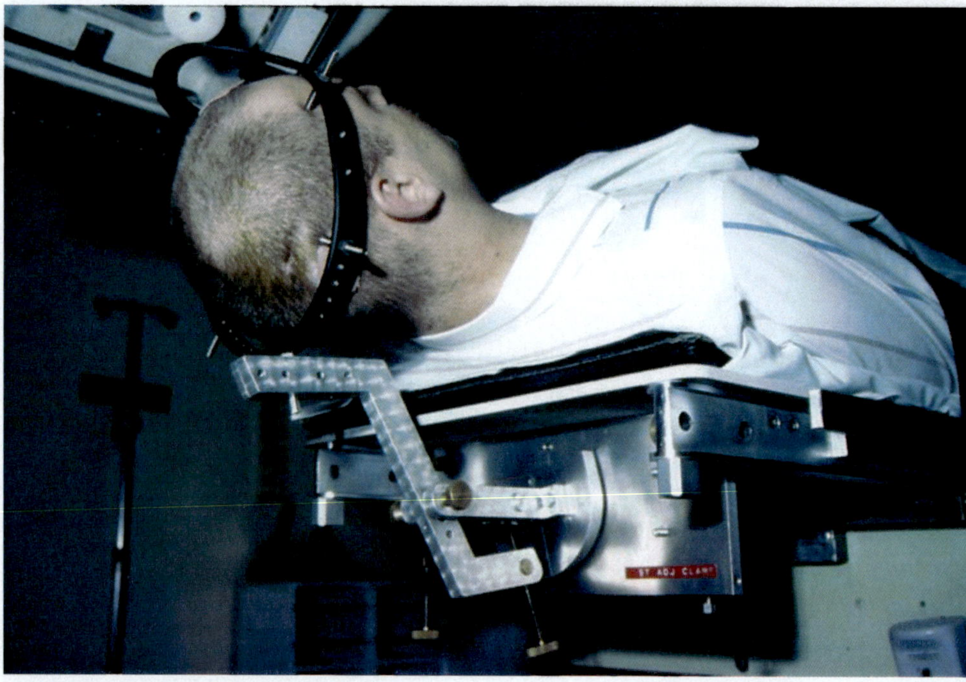

Figure 2: Immobilization halo ring.

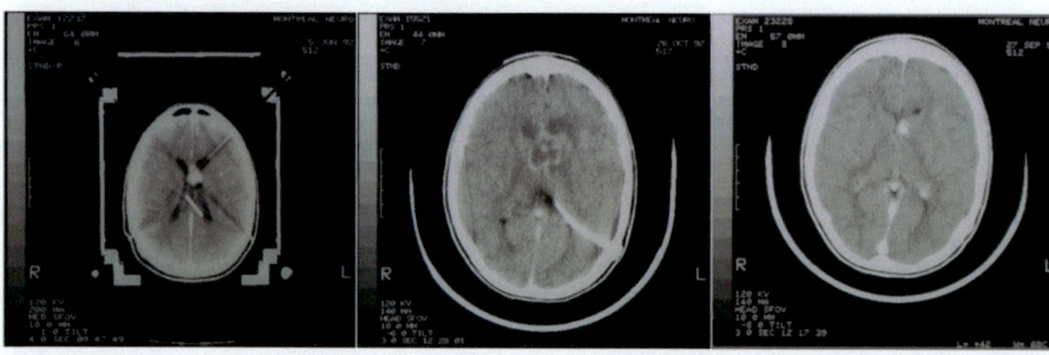

Figure 3: Grade II astrocytoma treated with F-SRT. At the age of 6, this young girl was diagnosed with tuberous sclerosis following an investigation for seizures. At the age of 11, through a transcallosal approach, she underwent subtotal resection of a growing left septum pellucidum lesion. On pathology, this was a grade II astrocytoma. The residual tumor was treated with F-SRT to a dose of 42 Gy in 6 fractions over 2 weeks (left). Four months later the center of the lesion became hypodense (center) before shrinking (right). The patient has been free of progression with a stable radiological abnormality for more than 10 years.

With a median follow-up for living patients of 13.3 years, the actuarial 15-year overall survival is 63% (Figure I). In initial response to the treatment 7 patients had a decrease in size of their tumor (33%), 5 had stable disease (24%) and a total of 9 patients (43%) have shown clear evidence of disease progression. The case of a patient with a favorable outcome following treatment with the fractionated regimen is presented in Figure III. Responses to treatment were clearly heterogeneous as demonstrated by patients with rapid post-therapy progression (see Figure 4) more typical of high-grade gliomas. In some of these cases it may be that stereotactic biopsy failed to sample a more histologically aggressive tumor component.

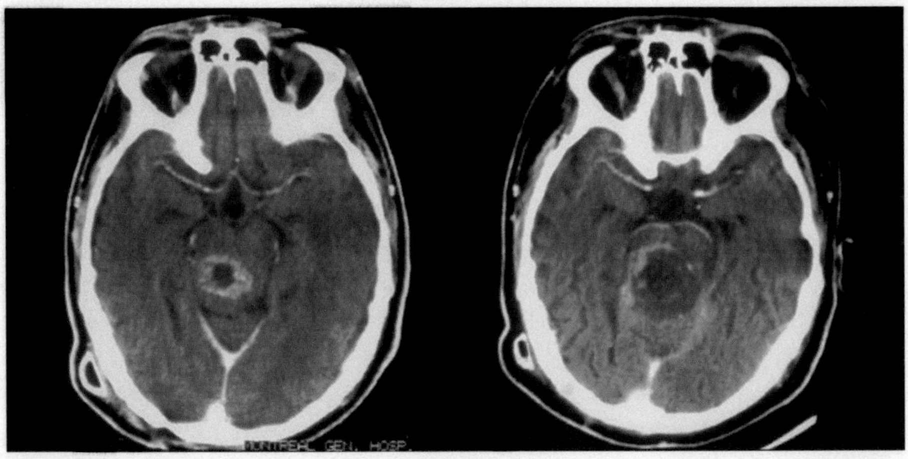

Figure 4: Treatment failure of histologically grade II astrocytoma treated with F-SRT. This 27-year-old patient was diagnosed with a grade II astrocytoma by stereotactic biopsy. He was treated with F-SRT (42 Gy in 6 fractions). The tumor progressed within months and the patient died exactly 1 year post therapy.

Treatment Toxicities

Significant acute complications – i.e., those occurring within days to weeks of treatment - are unusual and generally self-limited. Occasionally an exacerbation of existing symptoms may occur, particularly in patients with moderate brain edema and with larger lesions (3-4 cm). Most patients will respond to increasing doses of corticosteroids.

In our own series 3 patients had late complications post therapy. Ten months following F-SRT, a patient had transient symptoms of peri-lesional edema requiring steroids. A second patient had persistent worsening of his hemiparesis 4 months post-treatment. In the third case a patient had refractory edema 10 months post-treatment and was reoperated — at surgery both tumor and necrosis were seen.

Clark et al. [76], from McGill University, have described the determination of a single number parameter for use during F-SRT that may be used to represent effective dosage to intracranial structures that are irradiated with inhomogeneous dose distribution having steep dose gradients. Evaluating biologically effective dose volume histograms, the authors obtained an integral biologically effective dose (IBED) for each case and demonstrated a threshold value for late damage to the brain stem consistent with similar thresholds that have been determined for external beam radiation therapy. Using an α/β ratio of 2.5 as representative of the dose-response of brain stem tissue, they were able to establish a threshold value in the region of 60 $Gy_{2.5}$. The determination of the IBED can be a valuable parameter to be used as a guide to determine the appropriate treatment volume and fractionation regimen that will minimize toxicity to surrounding vital structures in patients undergoing F-SRT.

Often of more concern than focal brain injury is the risk of neurocognitive deficits following radiotherapy. In an attempt to quantify these risks, Folstein mini-mental state examination (MMSE) scores were reviewed for patients free of progressive tumor in the Intergroup dose-escalation trial [77]. With the caveat that the MMSE may be insensitive to subtle changes, only a small proportion of patients experienced a clinically significant decrease in their score from baseline. At years 1, 2 and 5, 8%, 5% and 5%, respectively, of patients experienced a significant decrease. Baseline variable, including radiation dose, conformal vs. conventional radiotherapy, number of fields, age, seizures and tumor size did not predict cognitive function change. Patients with baseline MMSE impairment actually had a greater probability of improvement than deterioration (59% vs. 12% at 1 year). It is interesting that there was a trend towards worse neurocognitive outcome in patients with tumors $\geq$ 5 cm ($p = 0.081$). In a series of adult brain tumor patients evaluated with a neuropsychological test battery emphasizing attention and concentration, Kaleita et al. [78] did not find a strong association between the use of radiotherapy and neurocognitive performance but did see a negative association with advanced age and frontal location of the tumor. In a cross-sectional study from the Netherlands involving 195 patients with low-grade gliomas (104 having received radiation) and 295 control patients, neurocopsychological testing was performed in four domains (memory, intelligence, attention and executive function, perception and psychomotor speed) [79]. Not surprisingly cognitive disability (as defined by the authors) was more common in the glioma patients than in controls with other low-grade malignancies (34% vs. 22%, $p = 0.035$). Cognitive disability was seen in patients whether or not they had received radiotherapy. In this case-control study, radiotherapy was associated with a higher risk of cognitive dysfunction but this was predominantly seen in patients treated with daily fractions of more than 2 Gy. It was the conclusion of the authors that conventionally fractionated radiation was not significantly associated with a worse cognitive outcome.

Children are known to be more sensitive to the deleterious effects of radiotherapy. Neurocognitive impairment has been well documented following whole brain radiotherapy for medulloblastoma or acute lymphocytic leukemia [80, 81]. There are several small retrospective series in which radiotherapy for low-grade tumors is associated with late neurocognitive dysfunction. As an example, in a series from Pollack et al. [82], 34% of patients with hemispheric astrocytomas treated with radiotherapy suffered from cognitive dysfunction. In reviewing this and other series [42, 83-88], young age and neurofibromatosis appear to be risk factors for late toxicity [89]. The risk of cognitive impairment may be lessened by modern radiotherapy techniques as reflected in series of conformal photon [90] or proton irradiation [91].

Although few of these patients have undergone formal neurocognitive testing, reports of late neurocognitive deficits following SRS are rare [92]. This is not unexpected in view of the small volumes treated and the steep dose fall-off.

Thorough neurocognitive measures will be available from recent Phase II trials [93, 94]. These measures will help better quantify the risk to the pediatric population treated with modern radiotherapy but will not discriminate the etiology of the deficits. The presence and magnitude of cognitive defects related to modern external beam radiotherapy being debated, it is difficult to quantify any gain which could be expected from the use of SRS — especially if irradiation of the same small targets would be compared to highly conformal external beam radiotherapy with tight margins and conventional (1.8-2.0 Gy daily) fractionation.

Discussion

When considering the theoretical advantages of SRS over conventional irradiation, it is of value to separate the different biological and technical issues, such as:

- The biology of single/large fractions;
- The reduced margins for both clinical and planning target volumes;
- The high dose conformality characteristic of stereotactic treatments.

Low-grade glioma is generally a local disease. Pattern of failure data was available for 65 of 114 patients who progressed on the Intergroup dose escalation trial. Of these 65 patients, 92% progressed within a 2 cm margin from the tumor edge [22]. In a report of 38 children treated for low-grade gliomas on a Phase II trial of conformal irradiation, 4 recurrences were reported [94]. Three were within the 10 mm clinical target volume margin and 1 patient had a failure adjacent to this margin. In a prospective trial of conventionally fractionated stereotactic radiotherapy, no marginal failures occurred despite the use of 2 mm margins [93]. As a high rate of disease-free survival is seen after complete resection of the radiologically defined tumor [24], it would appear reasonable to use reduced treatment margins. The minimally safe clinical target volume margin has yet to be defined but it is unrelated to the radiation modality used. On the other hand, the planning target volume is reduced in stereotactic techniques using rigid immobilization for which the set-up margin is generally 0 mm [73, 95]. However with advances in modern non-invasive patient immobilization systems and image-guidance, positioning reproducibility of 2 mm or less can routinely be achieved [96-98]. With the doses used for standard external beam therapy, it is unlikely that this extra 2 mm margin of normal brain will lead to significant late toxicity.

When SRS was first clinically implemented, it was not uncommon for conventionally-treated patients to be irradiated using low energy photons and parallel-opposed fields [44]. With technological advances in radiation therapy, the distinction between F-SRT and so-called conventional external beam radiotherapy is rapidly disappearing. When one compares the series of labeled "3D-CRT" from St-Jude Children's Research Hospital [94] to one labeled "fractionated stereotactic radiotherapy" from Dana-Farber [93], it is hard to identify any significant differences in dose distributions or immobilization. The main difference is in the margin selected by the physicians at these institutions (2 mm vs. 10 mm).

As discussed in the introduction, two randomized trials have failed to show any dose-response for low-grade gliomas in the range of 45-64.8 Gy [22, 45]. In contrast to high-grade gliomas, stereotactic irradiation has not been considered a means of dose escalation in so-called benign tumors. All other parameters being equal, single/large fractions are considered biologically disadvantageous for both normal tissue toxicity and tumor control [99]. An interesting hypothesis in the case of low-grade tumors, born of the known effects of SRS in vascular malformation, is that the larger fractions would act through an effect on tumor vasculature. Animal experiments with benign tumors have not clearly born this out [100].

In reviewing the current results of SRS and F-SRT, one could note that complete responses are rarely seen following conventional external beam therapy of adult low-grade gliomas. For 177 patients treated with external beam radiotherapy in a large randomized trial, the complete response rate was 2% [22]. Although the complete response rates for the retrospective series in this review certainly appear greater than 2%, one must remember the important biases favoring these series (namely size and age). In a series of 19 pediatric patients treated with conventional external beam radiotherapy at the London regional cancer center, the complete response rate was 21%. One must also keep in mind that radiological response may not correlate with clinical symptom improvement or survival [101, 102]. In reviewing these series, it is important remember the large numbers of patients with malignant gliomas treated with SRS [49] before a randomized trial confirmed concerns regarding the inherent biases of SRS series [56]. The outcomes of patients with low-grade gliomas are even more heterogeneous where subgroups can be defined where > 95% of patient survive their tumor [3] and subgroups where > 95% succumb to it [37]. It is thus not possible to draw any firm conclusions from small series with patients of mixed prognosis.

In our own experience, the 5-year survival of 69% in adult patients (none of the few pediatric patients died) was not strikingly different from what is expected in a cohort of young patients. Eighty percent of our adult patients were younger than 40 years of age, a subgroup with a 77% 5-year survival in the NCCTG dose trial [22]. Considering this lack of a clear therapeutic advantage we stopped using this FSRT scheme in late 1992.

Although a randomized trial would be required to properly define the role of SRS in low-grade glial tumors there is little enthusiasm for such an endeavor and realistically there may not be enough patients with small unresectable tumors to properly power such a trial. Illustrating this point, from July 1993 to October 1997 recurrent low-grade gliomas (and other metastatic, recurrent brain tumors) were eligible for SRS on a phase II study of the then Pediatric Oncology Group. The trial was planned to accrue 25 patients but closed early due to poor accrual. Only a total of 7 patients were treated on this protocol. The characteristics and outcomes of these patients have not been published. Of note, despite the conservative prescribing scheme (15 Gy prescribed to the 80% isodose surface using a single isocenter), 2/7 patients experienced grade 4 toxicity.

Current cooperative group interest lies in investigating the role of chemotherapy in the initial management of low-grade gliomas. The RTOG conducted a phase III of radiation with or without PCV chemotherapy for unfavorable low-grade glioma. This trial closed on June 27, 2002 after meeting its meeting accrual goal of 252 patients — results are pending. In January 2005, the RTOG opened a replacement Phase II trial evaluating a temozolomide-based chemo-radiotherapy regimen for high-risk low-grade gliomas. This Phase II regimen incorporates concurrent and adjuvant temozolomide with 54 Gy of conventional external beam radiotherapy. Only patients ≥ 40 years of age with preoperative tumor diameters ≥ 6 cm are eligible. An EORTC/NCIC trial will randomize patients between radiotherapy and protracted chemotherapy with oral temozolomide [103]. If concurrent chemo-radiotherapy is proven to be beneficial in low-grade tumors, the already limited number of patients considered for SRS will likely decrease even more.

Conclusion

Although the use of SRS for well-defined small low-grade tumors is appealing, the data regarding the use of SRS is limited and insufficient to support a standard role for SRS in the initial management of low-grade gliomas.

The technologies of F-SRT will slowly be integrated into conventional therapy, treatment margins will be reduced and SRS will be limited to very selected recurrent tumors.

References

[1] Surawicz TS, McCarthy BJ, Kupelian V, *et al.* Descriptive epidemiology of primary brain and CNS tumors: results from the Central Brain Tumor Registry of the United States, 1990-1994. *Neuro-oncol* 1999;1:14-25.

[2] Tumors of the Pediatric Central Nervous System. New York: Thieme; 2001.

[3] Dirven CM, Mooij JJ, Molenaar WM. Cerebellar pilocytic astrocytoma: a treatment protocol based upon analysis of 73 cases and a review of the literature. *Childs Nerv Syst* 1997;13:17-23.

[4] Due-Tonnessen BJ, Helseth E, Scheie D, *et al.* Long-term outcome after resection of benign cerebellar astrocytomas in children and young adults (0-19 years): report of 110 consecutive cases. *Pediatr Neurosurg* 2002;37:71-80.

[5] Gajjar A, Sanford RA, Heideman R, *et al.* Low-grade astrocytoma: a decade of experience at St. Jude Children's Research Hospital. *J Clin Oncol* 1997;15:2792-2799.

[6] Bauman G, Lote K, Larson D, *et al.* Pretreatment factors predict overall survival for patients with low-grade glioma: a recursive partitioning analysis. *Int J Radiat Oncol Biol Phys* 1999;45:923-929.

[7] Piepmeier J, Christopher S, Spencer D, *et al.* Variations in the natural history and survival of patients with supratentorial low-grade astrocytomas. *Neurosurgery* 1996;38:872-878; discussion 878-879.

[8] van Veelen ML, Avezaat CJ, Kros JM, *et al.* Supratentorial low grade astrocytoma: prognostic factors, dedifferentiation, and the issue of early versus late surgery. *J Neurol Neurosurg Psychiatry* 1998;64:581-587.

[9] Schuurman PR, Troost D, Verbeeten B, Jr., *et al.* 5-year survival and clinical prognostic factors in progressive supratentorial diffuse "low-grade" astrocytoma: a retrospective analysis of 46 cases. *Acta Neurochir (Wien)* 1997;139:2-7.

[10] Pignatti F, van den Bent M, Curran D, *et al.* Prognostic factors for survival in adult patients with cerebral low-grade glioma. *J Clin Oncol* 2002;20:2076-2084.

[11] Berger MS, Deliganis AV, Dobbins J, *et al.* The effect of extent of resection on recurrence in patients with low grade cerebral hemisphere gliomas. *Cancer* 1994;74:1784-1791.

[12] Lote K, Egeland T, Hager B, *et al.* Survival, prognostic factors, and therapeutic efficacy in low-grade glioma: a retrospective study in 379 patients. *J Clin Oncol* 1997;15:3129-3140.

[13] Desai KI, Nadkarni TD, Muzumdar DP, *et al.* Prognostic factors for cerebellar astrocytomas in children: a study of 102 cases. *Pediatr Neurosurg* 2001;35:311-317.

[14] Plathow C, Schulz-Ertner D, Thilman C, *et al.* Fractionated stereotactic radiotherapy in low-grade astrocytomas: long-term outcome and prognostic factors. *Int J Radiat Oncol Biol Phys* 2003;57:996-1003.

[15] Westergaard L, Gjerris F, Klinken L. Prognostic parameters in benign astrocytomas. *Acta Neurochir (Wien)* 1993;123:1-7.

[16] Franklin CI. The treatment of low grade cerebral astrocytomas by radiotherapy in Queensland. *Australas Radiol* 1991;35:68-71.

[17] Janny P, Cure H, Mohr M, *et al.* Low grade supratentorial astrocytomas. Management and prognostic factors. *Cancer* 1994;73:1937-1945.

[18] Lindegaard KF, Mork SJ, Eide GE, *et al.* Statistical analysis of clinicopathological features, radiotherapy, and survival in 170 cases of oligodendroglioma. *J Neurosurg* 1987;67:224-230.

[19] Stupp R, Janzer RC, Hegi ME, *et al.* Prognostic factors for low-grade gliomas. *Semin Oncol* 2003;30:23-28.

[20] Scott CB, Scarantino C, Urtasun R, *et al.* Validation and predictive power of Radiation Therapy Oncology Group (RTOG) recursive partitioning analysis classes for malignant glioma patients: a report using RTOG 90-06. *Int J Radiat Oncol Biol Phys* 1998;40:51-55.

[21] Curran WJ, Jr., Scott CB, Horton J, *et al.* Recursive partitioning analysis of prognostic factors in three Radiation Therapy Oncology Group malignant glioma trials. *J Natl Cancer Inst* 1993;85:704-710.

[22] Shaw E, Arusell R, Scheithauer B, *et al.* Prospective randomized trial of low- versus high-dose radiation therapy in adults with supratentorial low-grade glioma: initial report of a North Central Cancer Treatment Group/Radiation Therapy Oncology Group/Eastern Cooperative Oncology Group study. *J Clin Oncol* 2002;20:2267-2276.

[23] Kreth FW, Faist M, Rossner R, *et al.* Supratentorial World Health Organization Grade 2 astrocytomas and oligoastrocytomas. A new pattern of prognostic factors. *Cancer* 1997;79:370-379.

[24] Wisoff JH, Sanford A, Holmes E, *et al.* Impact of surgical resection on low grade gliomas of childhood: A report from the CCG9891/POG9130 low grade astrocytoma study. *Proc Am Soc Clin Oncol* 2003;22:100 (abstr 401).

[25] Laws ER, Jr. Resection of low-grade gliomas. *J Neurosurg* 2001;95:731-732.

[26] Rajan B, Pickuth D, Ashley S, *et al.* The management of histologically unverified presumed cerebral gliomas with radiotherapy. *Int J Radiat Oncol Biol Phys* 1994;28:405-413.

[27] Stieber VW. Low-grade gliomas. *Curr Treat Options Oncol* 2001;2:495-506.

[28] Freeman CR, Farmer JP, Montes J. Low-grade astrocytomas in children: evolving management strategies. *Int J Radiat Oncol Biol Phys* 1998;41:979-987.

[29] Gjerris F, Klinken L. Long-term prognosis in children with benign cerebellar astrocytoma. *J Neurosurg* 1978;49:179-184.

[30] Mercuri S, Russo A, Palma L. Hemispheric supratentorial astrocytomas in children. Long-term results in 29 cases. *J Neurosurg* 1981;55:170-173.

[31] Hirsch JF, Sainte Rose C, Pierre-Kahn A, *et al.* Benign astrocytic and oligodendrocytic tumors of the cerebral hemispheres in children. *J Neurosurg* 1989;70:568-572.

[32] Conway PD, Oechler HW, Kun LE, *et al.* Importance of histologic condition and treatment of pediatric cerebellar astrocytoma. *Cancer* 1991;67:2772-2775.

[33] Soffietti R, Chio A, Giordana MT, *et al.* Prognostic factors in well-differentiated cerebral astrocytomas in the adult. *Neurosurgery* 1989;24:686-692.

[34] Laws ER, Jr., Taylor WF, Clifton MB, *et al.* Neurosurgical management of low-grade astrocytoma of the cerebral hemispheres. *J Neurosurg* 1984;61:665-673.

[35] Medbery CA, 3rd, Straus KL, Steinberg SM, *et al.* Low-grade astrocytomas: treatment results and prognostic variables. *Int J Radiat Oncol Biol Phys* 1988;15:837-841.

[36] Shaw EG, Scheithauer BW, O'Fallon JR, *et al.* Mixed oligoastrocytomas: a survival and prognostic factor analysis. *Neurosurgery* 1994;34:577-582; discussion 582.

[37] North CA, North RB, Epstein JA, *et al.* Low-grade cerebral astrocytomas. Survival and quality of life after radiation therapy. *Cancer* 1990;66:6-14.

[38] Eyre HJ, Crowley JJ, Townsend JJ, *et al.* A randomized trial of radiotherapy versus radiotherapy plus CCNU for incompletely resected low-grade gliomas: a Southwest Oncology Group study. *J Neurosurg* 1993;78:909-914.

[39] Cairncross G, Seiferheld W, Shaw E, *et al.* An intergroup randomized controlled clinical trial (RCT) of chemotherapy plus radiation (RT) versus RT alone for pure and mixed anaplastic oligodendrogliomas: Initial report of RTOG 94-02. *Journal of Clinical Oncology, 2004 ASCO Annual Meeting Proceedings (Post-Meeting Edition)* 2004;22:1500.

[40] Buckner JC, Gesme D, Jr., O'Fallon JR, *et al.* Phase II trial of procarbazine, lomustine, and vincristine as initial therapy for patients with low-grade oligodendroglioma or oligoastrocytoma: efficacy and associations with chromosomal abnormalities. *J Clin Oncol* 2003;21:251-255.

[41] Stege EM, Kros JM, de Bruin HG, *et al.* Successful treatment of low-grade oligodendroglial tumors with a chemotherapy regimen of procarbazine, lomustine, and vincristine. *Cancer* 2005;103:802-809.

[42] Janss AJ, Grundy R, Cnaan A, *et al.* Optic pathway and hypothalamic/chiasmatic gliomas in children younger than age 5 years with a 6-year follow-up. *Cancer* 1995;75:1051-1059.

[43] Elvidge AR. Long-term survival in the astrocytoma series. *J Neurosurg* 1968;28:399-404.

[44] Bouchard J. Radiation Therapy of Tumors and Diseases of the Nervous System. Philadelphia: Lea and Febiger; 1966.

[45] Karim AB, Maat B, Hatlevoll R, *et al.* A randomized trial on dose-response in radiation therapy of low-grade cerebral glioma: European Organization for Research and Treatment of Cancer (EORTC) Study 22844. *Int J Radiat Oncol Biol Phys* 1996;36:549-556.

[46] Karim AB, Afra D, Cornu P, *et al.* Randomized trial on the efficacy of radiotherapy for cerebral low-grade glioma in the adult: European Organization for Research and Treatment of Cancer Study 22845 with the Medical Research Council study BRO4: an interim analysis. *Int J Radiat Oncol Biol Phys* 2002;52:316-324.

[47] Shaw EG, Tatter SB, Lesser GJ, *et al.* Current controversies in the radiotherapeutic management of adult low-grade glioma. *Semin Oncol* 2004;31:653-658.

[48] Leksell L. The stereotaxic method and radiosurgery of the brain. *Acta chirurgica Scandinavia* 1951;102:316-319.

[49] Roberge D, Souhami L. Stereotactic radiosurgery in the management of intracranial gliomas. *Technol Cancer Res Treat* 2003;2:117-125.

[50] Wallner KE, Galicich JH, Krol G, *et al.* Patterns of failure following treatment for glioblastoma multiforme and anaplastic astrocytoma. *Int J Radiat Oncol Biol Phys* 1989;16:1405-1409.

[51] Gutin PH, Prados MD, Phillips TL, *et al.* External irradiation followed by an interstitial high activity iodine-125 implant "boost" in the initial treatment of malignant gliomas: NCOG study 6G-82-2. *Int J Radiat Oncol Biol Phys* 1991;21:601-606.

[52] Loeffler JS, Alexander E, 3rd, Hochberg FH, *et al.* Clinical patterns of failure following stereotactic interstitial irradiation for malignant gliomas. *Int J Radiat Oncol Biol Phys* 1990;19:1455-1462.

[53] Kondziolka D, Flickinger JC, Bissonette DJ, *et al.* Survival benefit of stereotactic radiosurgery for patients with malignant glial neoplasms. *Neurosurgery* 1997;41:776-783; discussion 783-775.

[54] Irish WD, Macdonald DR, Cairncross JG. Measuring bias in uncontrolled brain tumor trials--to randomize or not to randomize? *Can J Neurol Sci* 1997;24:307-312.

[55] Lustig RA, Scott CB, Curran WJ. Does stereotactic eligibility for the treatment of glioblastoma cause selection bias in randomized studies? *Am J Clin Oncol* 2004;27:516-521.

[56] Souhami L, Seiferheld W, Brachman D, *et al.* Randomized comparison of stereotactic radiosurgery followed by conventional radiotherapy with carmustine to conventional radiotherapy with carmustine for patients with glioblastoma multiforme: report of Radiation Therapy Oncology Group 93-05 protocol. *Int J Radiat Oncol Biol Phys* 2004;60:853-860.

[57] Zietman AL, Suit HD, Tomkinson KN, *et al.* The response of two human tumor xenografts to fractionated irradiation. The derivation of alpha/beta ratios from growth delay, tumor control, and in vitro cell survival assays. *Int J Radiat Oncol Biol Phys* 1990;18:569-575.

[58] Marin LA, Smith CE, Langston MY, *et al.* Response of glioblastoma cell lines to low dose rate irradiation. *Int J Radiat Oncol Biol Phys* 1991;21:397-402.

[59] Raza SM, Lang FF, Aggarwal BB, *et al.* Necrosis and glioblastoma: a friend or a foe? A review and a hypothesis. *Neurosurgery* 2002;51:2-12; discussion 12-13.

[60] Stuschke M, Budach V, Sack H. Radioresponsiveness of human glioma, sarcoma, and breast cancer spheroids depends on tumor differentiation. *Int J Radiat Oncol Biol Phys* 1993;27:627-636.

[61] Kondziolka D, Lunsford LD, Flickinger JC. Stereotactic Radiosurgery. In: Keating RF, Goodrich JT, Packer RJ, editors. Tumors of the Pediatric Central Nervous System. New York: Thieme; 2001. p. 560.

[62] Colombo F, Benedetti A, Pozza F, *et al.* External stereotactic irradiation by linear accelerator. *Neurosurgery* 1985;16:154-160.

[63] Pozza F, Colombo F, Chierego G, *et al.* Low-grade astrocytomas: treatment with unconventionally fractionated external beam stereotactic radiation therapy. *Radiology* 1989;171:565-569.

[64] Barcia JA, Barcia-Salorio JL, Ferrer C, *et al.* Stereotactic radiosurgery of deeply seated low grade gliomas. *Acta Neurochir Suppl* 1994;62:58-61.

[65] Kida Y, Kobayashi T, Mori Y. Gamma knife radiosurgery for low-grade astrocytomas: results of long-term follow up. *J Neurosurg* 2000;93 Suppl 3:42-46.

[66] Hadjipanayis CG, Kondziolka D, Gardner P, *et al.* Stereotactic radiosurgery for pilocytic astrocytomas when multimodal therapy is necessary. *J Neurosurg* 2002;97:56-64.

[67] Hadjipanayis CG, Kondziolka D, Flickinger JC, *et al.* The role of stereotactic radiosurgery for low-grade astrocytomas. *Neurosurg Focus* 2003;14:e15.

[68] Hadjipanayis CG, Niranjan A, Tyler-Kabara E, *et al.* Stereotactic radiosurgery for well-circumscribed fibrillary grade II astrocytomas: an initial experience. *Stereotact Funct Neurosurg* 2002;79:13-24.

[69] Boethius J, Ulfarsson E, Rahn T, *et al.* Gamma knife radiosurgery for pilocytic astrocytomas. *J Neurosurg* 2002;97:677-680.

[70] Simonova G, Novotny J, Jr., Liscak R. Low-grade gliomas treated by fractionated gamma knife surgery. *J Neurosurg* 2005;102 Suppl:19-24.

[71] Olivier A, Peters T, Bertrand G. Stereotactic system and apparatus for use with magnetic resonance imaging, computerized tomography, and digital subtraction imaging. *Appl Neurophysiol* 1985;48:94-96.

[72] Peters TM, Clark JA, Olivier A, *et al.* Integrated stereotaxic imaging with CT, MR imaging, and digital subtraction angiography. *Radiology* 1986;161:821-826.

[73] Clark BG, Podgorsak EB, Souhami L, *et al.* A halo-ring technique for fractionated stereotactic radiotherapy. *Br J Radiol* 1993;66:522-527.

[74] Podgorsak EB, Olivier A, Pla M, *et al.* Dynamic stereotactic radiosurgery. *Int J Radiat Oncol Biol Phys* 1988;14:115-126.

[75] Podgorsak EB, Souhami L, Caron JL, *et al.* A technique for fractionated stereotactic radiotherapy in the treatment of intracranial tumors. *Int J Radiat Oncol Biol Phys* 1993;27:1225-1230.

[76] Clark BG, Souhami L, Pla C, *et al.* The integral biologically effective dose to predict brain stem toxicity of hypofractionated stereotactic radiotherapy. *Int J Radiat Oncol Biol Phys* 1998;40:667-675.

[77] Brown PD, Buckner JC, O'Fallon JR, *et al.* Effects of radiotherapy on cognitive function in patients with low-grade glioma measured by the folstein mini-mental state examination. *J Clin Oncol* 2003;21:2519-2524.

[78] Kaleita TA, Wellisch DK, Cloughesy TF, *et al.* Prediction of neurocognitive outcome in adult brain tumor patients. *J Neurooncol* 2004;67:245-253.

[79] Klein M, Heimans JJ, Aaronson NK, *et al.* Effect of radiotherapy and other treatment-related factors on mid-term to long-term cognitive sequelae in low-grade gliomas: a comparative study. *Lancet* 2002;360:1361-1368.

[80] Mulhern RK, Fairclough D, Ochs J. A prospective comparison of neuropsychologic performance of children surviving leukemia who received 18-Gy, 24-Gy, or no cranial irradiation. *J Clin Oncol* 1991;9:1348-1356.

[81] Mulhern RK, Kepner JL, Thomas PR, *et al.* Neuropsychologic functioning of survivors of childhood medulloblastoma randomized to receive conventional or reduced-dose craniospinal irradiation: a Pediatric Oncology Group study. *J Clin Oncol* 1998;16:1723-1728.

[82] Pollack IF, Claassen D, al-Shboul Q, *et al.* Low-grade gliomas of the cerebral hemispheres in children: an analysis of 71 cases. *J Neurosurg* 1995;82:536-547.

[83] Danoff BF, Cowchock FS, Marquette C, *et al.* Assessment of the long-term effects of primary radiation therapy for brain tumors in children. *Cancer* 1982;49:1580-1586.

[84] Lloyd LA. Gliomas of the optic nerve and chiasm in childhood. *Trans Am Ophthalmol Soc* 1973;71:488-535.

[85] Rodriguez LA, Edwards MS, Levin VA. Management of hypothalamic gliomas in children: an analysis of 33 cases. *Neurosurgery* 1990;26:242-246; discussion 246-247.

[86] Sutton LN, Molloy PT, Sernyak H, *et al.* Long-term outcome of hypothalamic/chiasmatic astrocytomas in children treated with conservative surgery. *J Neurosurg* 1995;83:583-589.

[87] Tao ML, Barnes PD, Billett AL, *et al.* Childhood optic chiasm gliomas: radiographic response following radiotherapy and long-term clinical outcome. *Int J Radiat Oncol Biol Phys* 1997;39:579-587.

[88] Weiss L, Sagerman RH, King GA, *et al.* Controversy in the management of optic nerve glioma. *Cancer* 1987;59:1000-1004.

[89] Kortmann RD, Timmermann B, Taylor RE, *et al.* Current and future strategies in radiotherapy of childhood low-grade glioma of the brain. Part II: Treatment-related late toxicity. *Strahlenther Onkol* 2003;179:585-597.

[90] Saran FH, Baumert BG, Khoo VS, *et al.* Stereotactically guided conformal radiotherapy for progressive low-grade gliomas of childhood. *Int J Radiat Oncol Biol Phys* 2002;53:43-51.

[91] Hug EB, Muenter MW, Archambeau JO, *et al.* Conformal proton radiation therapy for pediatric low-grade astrocytomas. *Strahlenther Onkol* 2002;178:10-17.

[92] McDonald CR, Norman MA, Tecoma E, *et al.* Neuropsychological change following gamma knife surgery in patients with left temporal lobe epilepsy: a review of three cases. *Epilepsy Behav* 2004;5:949-957.

[93] Marcus KJ, Goumnerova L, Billett AL, *et al.* Stereotactic radiotherapy for localized low-grade gliomas in children: final results of a prospective trial. *Int J Radiat Oncol Biol Phys* 2005;61:374-379.

[94] Merchant TE, Zhu Y, Thompson SJ, *et al.* Preliminary results from a Phase II trail of conformal radiation therapy for pediatric patients with localised low-grade astrocytoma and ependymoma. *Int J Radiat Oncol Biol Phys* 2002;52:325-332.

[95] MacKenzie JT, Podgorsak MB, Moreland D. Validity of stereotactic frame localization during radiosurgery after one fixation pin removal. *J Neurosurg* 2002;97:539-541.

[96] Alheit H, Dornfeld S, Dawel M, *et al.* Patient position reproducibility in fractionated stereotactically guided conformal radiotherapy using the BrainLab mask system. *Strahlenther Onkol* 2001;177:264-268.

[97] Burton KE, Thomas SJ, Whitney D, *et al.* Accuracy of a relocatable stereotactic radiotherapy head frame evaluated by use of a depth helmet. *Clin Oncol (R Coll Radiol)* 2002;14:31-39.

[98] Ryken TC, Meeks SL, Pennington EC, *et al.* Initial clinical experience with frameless stereotactic radiosurgery: analysis of accuracy and feasibility. *Int J Radiat Oncol Biol Phys* 2001;51:1152-1158.

[99] Brenner DJ, Martel MK, Hall EJ. Fractionated regimens for stereotactic radiotherapy of recurrent tumors in the brain. *Int J Radiat Oncol Biol Phys* 1991;21:819-824.

[100] Larson DA, Flickinger JC, Loeffler JS. The radiobiology of radiosurgery. *Int J Radiat Oncol Biol Phys* 1993;25:557-561.

[101] Fisher BJ, Bauman GS, Leighton CE, *et al.* Low-grade gliomas in children: tumor volume response to radiation. *J Neurosurg* 1998;88:969-974.

[102] Bauman G, Pahapill P, Macdonald D, *et al.* Low grade glioma: a measuring radiographic response to radiotherapy. *Can J Neurol Sci* 1999;26:18-22.

[103] Stupp R, Baumert BG. Promises and controversies in the management of low-grade glioma. *Ann Oncol* 2003;14:1695-1696.

[104] Pathology and Genetics of Tumors of the Nervous System. Lyon: IARCPress; 2000.

[105] Regine WF, Patchell RA, Strottmann JM, *et al.* Preliminary report of a phase I study of combined fractionated stereotactic radiosurgery and conventional external beam radiation therapy for unfavorable gliomas. *Int J Radiat Oncol Biol Phys* 2000;48:421-426.

Index

A

B

C

D

E

F

G

H

I

K

L

M

N

O

P

Q

R

S

U

V

W

X

Y

Z